# Combat Syndrome X, Y and Z...

OBESITY

HIGH BLOOD
PRESSURE

SYNDROME X ——— Y ——————— Z...

(Primary
cardiovascular risks,
heart attack,
coronary heart
disease and stroke)

(Blood clotting,
female endocrine
disorders, immune
impairment,
polycystic ovaries,
fatty liver)

(Eicosanoid
change with
inflammation
and cancer,
liver disease)

INSULIN
RESISTANCE

HIGH BLOOD
CHOLESTEROL

By

## Stephen Holt, M.D.

www.wellnesspublishing.com

# Combat Syndrome X, Y and Z...

WITHIN THE SYNDROME, X, Y AND Z,
THE X, Y AND Z ARE COMPOSED OF:

## X: THE VARIABLE COMBINATION OF:

- OBESITY
- HIGH BLOOD CHOLESTEROL
- INSULIN RESISTANCE
- HIGH BLOOD PRESSURE

## X: OUTCOMES

- PRIMARY CARDIOVASCULAR RISKS

## Y AND Z: THE VARIABLE COMBINATION OF:

- TENDENCY TO BLOOD CLOTTING
- FEMALE ENDOCRINE DISORDERS
- INFERTILITY
- IMPAIRED IMMUNITY
- EICOSANOID CHANGE
- INFLAMMATION AND CANCER?
- LIVER DISEASE
- POLYCYSTIC OVARIES

## Y, Z: OUTCOMES

- PROTEAN MANIFESTATIONS OF DISEASE

By

## Stephen Holt MD

Address questions to:
Review: www.combatsyndromeX.com
Email: info@combatsyndromeX.com

Manufactured in the United States.

Book and Cover Design: Jonathan Gullery

Library of Congress Cataloging-in-Publication Data.
Stephen Holt MD 1950-
COMBAT SYNDROME X, Y AND Z....
Stephen Holt MD (author) with forewords by Julian Whitaker MD and Jeff VanDrunen.
Includes biographical references and bibliography.
ISBN - 0-9714224-2-7
1. The Metabolic Syndrome 2. Syndrome X 3. Nutritional Medicine
4. Alternative Medicine 5. Lifestyle Changes 6. Diabetes mellitus
7. Obesity 8. Hypertension 9. Blood Cholesterol 10. Insulin Resistance 11.
Weight Control 12. Natural Products 13. Soluble Fiber
14. Unifying Concepts of Disease. I. Stephen Holt MD
II. COMBAT SYNDROME X, Y AND Z...., 2002

vwww. wellnesspublishing.com,
www.combatsyndromeX.com,
www.syndromeX.tv
www.sindromeX.com (in Spanish)
www.syndromeX.cc

# CONTENTS

# A NOTE TO THE READER

Whilst the health benefits of nutrition and remedies of natural origin are reviewed in this book, it is not the intention of the author to provide an alternative to the orthodox physician/patient relationship. The author discusses positive lifestyle changes and the use of non-allopathic remedies. It is his intention to expand the dimensions of orthodox medicine. This book was not written to endorse the use of a specific product and the author and publisher do not accept any liability for the use of any agents or products mentioned in this book. This book represents the author's opinion of scientific literature and lay press and opinion differs among many people.

Before any individual self-medicates or makes a major lifestyle change, he or she is advised to seek the advice of a qualified health care professional.

The author encourages dialogue between doctor and patient.

# ACKNOWLEDGMENT

With love and thanks for the endurance and patience shown by my wife, Karin Holt-von Ah. Much dedication was required to complete this work.

# DEDICATION

To Arnold, please get better.

# FOREWORD

## by Julian Whitaker, M.D.

Syndrome X, the constellation of medical conditions that includes obesity, abnormal blood lipids, and hypertension, is growing in epidemic proportions and is now estimated to affect as many as 70 million Americans. Yet a disturbing number of them are unaware that they face this serious health challenge, which is a prime cause of cardiac deaths and disabilities.

Dr. Holt's book on Syndrome X—or, to quote his new concept, "Syndrome X, Y and Z..."—provides a timely and much needed look at this increasingly common problem. He further expands the parameters of Syndrome X to provide a unifying concept of chronic disease beyond coronary heart disease, heart attacks, and stroke.

I am particularly impressed by Dr. Holt's approach to the prevention and treatment of Syndrome X, Y, and Z. Eschewing the conventional approach of drugs and more drugs, he provides the reader with an arsenal of safe and effective "orthomolecular" tools. Orthomolecular medicine, as defined by the late and great Nobel Prize-winning scientist Linus Pauling, Ph.D., is the use of substances normally present in the body in varying doses to engender health and treat disease. Dietary interventions and nutritional supplements are examples of orthomolecular treatments, and they are the focus of Dr. Holt's—and my—treatment of "Syndrome X, Y and Z."

This book provides a lucid account of the genetic and lifestyle factors underlying Syndrome X, Y and Z. It is full of good advice on how to prevent and correct this threat to your health. Dr. Holt's work is relevant to all health-conscious Americans—and it gives practicing physicians a reminder of the importance of lifestyle change, behavior modification, and nutritional interventions to combat Syndrome X, Y and Z.

Julian Whitaker MD
February 2002

# FOREWORD

## by Jeff Van Drunen

The food industry has attempted to address the health of the nation in many ways and it has received its fair share of criticism, as the role of good nutrition for well-being becomes increasingly clear. Nowhere is the attempt to correct health more apparent than in the fight against. cardiovascular disease which remains the main cause of death and disability in Western society. Modern research in food and medical science has focused on important cardiovascular risk factors, including obesity, high blood cholesterol, diabetes (glucose intolerance or insulin resistance), adverse lifestyle and hypertension. This constellation of disorders has been termed Syndrome X, terminology that stresses the complex interplay of risks that threaten cardiovascular health and cause other diseases. Whilst drug treatments for the components of Syndrome X are widely touted, this disorder is linked to both lifestyle and hereditary factors. As Dr. Holt indicates, the approach to a lifestyle disorder may be more linked to positive lifestyle change rather than drug treatments. Of all lifestyle domains, Dr. Holt's focus on nutritional approaches to Syndrome X (the metabolic syndrome) is timely.

Dr. Stephen Holt asked me to write this foreword to his book because he felt that a perspective from the food industry would make his important messages on the metabolic syndrome (Syndrome X) more portable. I share Dr. Holt's belief that the food industry must be increasingly cross-fertilized with medical care, in order to achieve real advances in public health. As we enter this new millennium, attempts to impact cardiovascular disorders present the number one public health initiative in the US. It is with great pleasure that I provide my perspective on the importance of Dr. Stephen Holt's interpretation of Dr. Reaven's initial characterization of Syndrome X, expanded in a novel and elegant manner to include the innovative concepts of Syndrome X, Y and Z... (Holt's Syndrome).

We have become increasingly aware of the stubborn presence of adverse lifestyle in industrialized communities. Although hereditary predispositions may contribute to many diseases, adverse lifestyle, including poor nutritional habits, is causing premature death. My family has been in the agricultural industry for more than a century and we have evolved with the opinion that good agricultural practices, with improved techniques of food processing,  provide the basis of healthy foods. For two decades, my family has focused on a mission to research and develop food ingredients that have disease prevention and treatment properties. This area of food science has been referred to in popular jargon as "functional food". I prefer to see this situation as the Hippocratic concept of "food as medicine".

I am convinced that this area of agricultural practice could promote health and longevity. This has increased our desire to work with "nutritional innovators" like Dr. Holt. The work described in this book is truly novel and pioneering. In his research, Dr. Stephen Holt MD has facilitated the acceptance of many different types of food with medicinal value into medical practice. The results of his work are admirable and evident in his many books and articles on nutritional approaches to disease prevention and treatment.

My interests in Syndrome X were initially peaked by reading the work of Dr. Gerald Reaven MD from Stanford, California but as I researched the literature, I found a wealth of information on the properties of plant substances, especially soluble fiber in, the fight against diabetes mellitus, obesity and high blood cholesterol.In my literature review, I was particularly impressed by the work of Dr. Holt in the 1970's on the effects of soluble fiber on upper gastrointestinal function, published in the Lancet in 1979. This work formed the basis of the understanding of what is now termed the Glycemic Index, a phrase coined in the 1980's by Dr. D. Jenkins MD of Toronto.

The public's increasing disenchantment with standard drug therapy for several life–threatening disorders has spurred my colleagues and I to further examine the development of functional food products which could be applied to help correct these problems in a simple and safe manner. The message in this book on the application of "food as medicine" could easily be missed, but some truly exciting biochemical research studies reveal how complex the beneficial effects of certain foods may be in the promotion of healthy body chemistry. This chemistry is the basis of the maintenance of healthy body structures and functions.

Stephen Holt MD identifies and provides interventional advice to combat Syndrome X, a medical catastrophe that effects tens of millions of Americans. Syndrome X is part of a hidden epidemic in Western society that includes the variable combination of insulin resistance, high blood pressure or cholesterol and obesity. In order to overcome the complacency that exists in trying to get people to correct adverse lifestyle that causes and propagates Syndrome X and ensuing cardiovascular disease, Dr. Holt has simplified complex scientific findings so that these common and serious health issues can be communicated to everyone. With the revelation that many healthcare professionals may have forgotten several natural options to combat cardiovascular disease, this work uncovers the disadvantages of a focus on single risk factors for cardiovascular health, at the expense of considering all risks together. To quote Dr. Holt, one must address the "bouquet of barbed wire" of cardiovascular risk factors.

Modern research shows us that Mother Nature has provided some simple ways to defeat Syndrome X. A striking feature of this book is the validity of its discussion about natural medicine and the revelation of the "secrets of soluble fiber" and other botanicals that can make a difference in the prevention and progression of Syndrome X, Y and Z.... Dr. Holt is to be credited with the explanation of the basis of the physiological effects of soluble fiber glucose absorption in humans. His research was published in the medical literature three years prior to the description of the Glycemic Index. In fact, Dr. Holt's early observations on the slowing of glucose absorption by the slowing of gastric emptying induced by soluble fiber, contribute greatly to our understanding of the "Glycemic Index" of foods. This book takes a second look at the "Glycemic Index" and makes the painstaking quantitation of the individual calculations of the glycemic index of different foods somewhat redundant.

This book extends the concepts about the value of soluble fiber by describing the intrinsic metabolic effects of fiber (IMEF) and it reveals how the end products of the metabolism of certain extracts of soluble oat fiber (short chain fatty acids, SCFA) act on the chemistry of the body to promote lowering of blood cholesterol and appetite reduction. The discussions in this book are supported by an expert appraisal of contemporary scientific literature and Dr. Holt broadens the concept of Syndrome X to what he terms "Syndrome X, Y and Z...Not only does this book examine healthy, natural options for the person with established coronary heart disease, it provides many other common-sense tactics for cardiovascular disease prevention, whilst acknowledging the value of conventional medical interventions. By expert navigation of scientific literature, Dr. Holt supports his notion of the existence of Syndrome X, Y and Z... with its wide ranging health risks.

In my own research, I have been interested in the medical use of fractions of soluble fiber manufactured from oats. Once considered relatively inert substances, dietary fibers have powerful health benefits on the body that are exerted in a complex manner. My family and I at Van Drunen Farms and our corporation Futureceuticals Inc. are engaged in the research of bulk food production by isolating fractions of plants and botanicals that have promising health benefits in the combat against Syndrome X.

Whilst Dr. Holt provided us with an explanation of how soluble fiber exerted its effects on blood glucose balance in the 1970's, he reviews the information on how fractions of soluble fiber result in end-products that act on the body in similar manner to drugs. This is part of the intrinsic metabolic effect of fiber (IMEF). Of particular importance is Dr. Holt's observation of the inhibition of HMG CoA-reductase in the liver by the end products of beta glucan fermentation in the colon (proprionic acid and other short chain fatty acids). These short chain fatty acids reach the liver by the blood stream where they exert several effects, including the lowering of blood cholesterol.. Who would have thought that something so apparently inert as soluble fiber could actually act like a "statin-type" cholesterol lowering drug by interfering with enzymes that control the synthesis of cholesterol in the liver? Dr. Holt had spoken about the "intrinsic metabolic effects" (IMEF) of fiber thirty years ago and this concept is still waiting to be further researched and applied. This book provides material to justify a major renaissance in interest in the versatile benefits of soluble fiber, especially the beta glucan fractions of oat fiber.

Of great interest is Dr. Holt's description of Syndrome X, Y and Z... He has expanded the concepts of "Dr. Reaven's Syndrome X" by defining how the central underlying problem of insulin resistance changes body chemistry in a manner that favors the development of several different diseases, including infertility and the polycystic ovary syndrome in young females and tendencies to develop blood clotting, cancer and inflammatory disorders. Dr. Holt's lateral thinking is beginning to "fill in" the picture puzzle on how nutritional building blocks can impact the principal public health concerns of our nation.

The concept of combining dietary adjustments and positive lifestyle changes; with the appropriate selection of nutritional options, distinguish the discussions in this book. Dr. Holt pioneers the expansion of what he terms "pluralistic medicine" in tackling the components of Syndrome X. The contribution of this book to the war against insulin resistance, with its association of high blood cholesterol, hypertension, obesity and cardiovascular disease is timely and powerful.  It is time to "Combat Syndrome X (of Reaven) or X, Y and Z... (of Holt)"

Jeff Van Drunen, December 2001
President, Futureceuticals Inc. and
Van Drunen Farms, Momence, Illinois

# PREFACE

What are we to do with the common but "occult" disorder called Syndrome X? Syndrome X affects up to 70 million Americans without widespread recognition of its presence, among its victims or their doctors. The term Syndrome X is applied to the variable combination of obesity, high blood cholesterol, poor blood glucose balance (insulin resistance) and high blood pressure. In its classic form, Syndrome X is characterized by the pot-bellied, fifty year-old person who worries about his or her blood cholesterol, whilst they are unaware of glucose intolerance due to insulin resistance. However, Syndrome X comes in many guises that share a common underlying feature of resistance to the actions of the hormone insulin. The constellation of disorders within Syndrome X aggregate together to kill or cripple many people in an insidious manner by creating a widespread risk for cardiovascular and other diseases. The title of this book expands the view of Reaven's Syndrome X into Syndrome X, Y and Z…, supported by the increasingly defined role of insulin resistance in the cause of female infertility, inflammatory disorders, immune impairment and perhaps cancer. Given the "health terrorism" that exists within the boundaries of Syndrome X, this book calls for "combat" against this common killer combination of disorders.

In popular language, we apply a qualification with the letter X when something is mysterious, provocative, sinister and perhaps unexplainable, e.g. X-Files, X-Men, Generation X and X-Rated. These qualities apply to syndrome X which is a sinister collection of causes of ill health and premature loss of life. Perhaps Syndrome X is best labeled the X-Degeneration of our younger generations. The cause and effect relationships among the four cardinal components of Syndrome X have become increasingly clear to modern science, largely as a consequence of the work of the eminent Stanford University physician, Dr. G. Reaven MD. Dr. Reaven coined the terms "Syndrome X" in 1988 to describe the interrelationship of obesity, high blood pressure and raised blood sugar (insulin resistance) with elevated blood cholesterol. Obesity was not featured strongly in Dr. Reaven's original hypothesis concerning Syndrome X, but there is clear evidence to incriminate "central-types" of obesity and perhaps changes of protein metabolism with high blood uric acid within the syndrome. In this book, I extend the observations further to support my notion of Syndrome X, Y and Z.... where disease risks beyond cardiovascular problems emerge with clarity. The disorders within Syndrome X are inextricably linked with adverse lifestyle in a "bouquet of barbed wire" that is both killing Western nations and robbing them of health.

There has been a tendency to ignore the need to impact "all" of the combined cardiovascular health risk factors that threaten mature individuals. It is now quite scary to identify these risks as operating increasingly in childhood. Faced with an epidemic of obesity, high blood cholesterol, glucose intolerance (insulin resistance or diabetes mellitus) and hypertension (the components of Syndrome X), much complacency still exists. Whilst the variable combination of the status of being fat, hypertensive, diabetic or prediabetic with hypercholesterolemia has been linked to cardiovascular disease, this combination of problems seems to have other far reaching health consequences affecting the occurrence of cancer, infertility and chronic inflammatory disease. This extended risk of Syndrome X beyond cardiovascular disease is described in this book as "Syndrome X, Y and Z...". This evil epidemic may affect more than one quarter of our population and it is a growing problem.

There are up to 20 million Americans with diabetes mellitus. Many do not know that they have it and there are many more who have a "pre-diabetic state". In August 2001, the U.S. Secretary of Human Health and Social Services joined researchers from Harvard University and the National Institutes of Health to call for a major public health initiative to educate the US population on the prevention of diabetes mellitus (and related disorders that form Syndrome X). These recent national proclamations warned of the shocking increase in diabetes and pre-diabetic disorders in all age groups and presented clear evidence that weight loss and exercise prevents these diseases. In a recent national TV broadcast (August, 2001), prominent researchers and government officials were not "beating a high technology drum" with new drugs or medical procedures, they were largely discussing the benefits of positive lifestyle change, including nutritional interventions. The tragic events of September 11th, 2001 temporarily took our national focus away from this important public health initiative, but Syndrome X is more damaging to our well-being than any foreseeable international conflict. Syndrome X is an ultimate form of bioterrorism, encouraged by the "Western lifestyle".

Whilst people are tired of being told that they are fat, sedentary and developing diabetes, many individuals have a health status rather like a "ticking time bomb". Many people with Syndrome X are ready to explode with a heart attack or other manifestations of cardiovascular disease. Scientific data, reported in Scotland, UK as recently as November 2001, shows that the increasing prevalence of diabetes has produced an eight fold increase in risks for heart disease. Furthermore, several other chronic diseases incubate in the individual with Syndrome X. Too many people in Western Society still recline whilst watching TV and "gobble" billions of dollars worth of "fast" or "junk food". Excessive amounts of refined sugar, saturated fat and salt with a deficiency of healthy fats and fiber in our diet is triggering Syndrome X. Our "fast food nation" recognizes the problem, but they seem to do little to change these destructive habits. In this book, I call for greater motivation to combat Syndrome X by addressing lifestyle issues, especially the nutritional and dietary habits of our nation.

The social, political and economic factors that determine our continuing adverse lifestyle are highly complex. The lure of fast food, with its clear cost- advantages, tend to overcome an individual's consideration of their health status. Children are mesmerized by fast food, indoctrinated by advertising and highly accepting of the established "sweet and fat" taste preference of industrialized society. "Happy meals" reward a child with a toy for eating fried food with a high saturated fat content. Adults share these temptations. It is known that degenerative disease often has its roots in childhood and we have bred a "mindset" in society where chronic debility is an accepted status for much of our elderly population. Recent evidence, however, shows that the occurrence of age-related, chronic degenerative diseases has been brought forward to childhood. These circumstances are obvious with reports of increasing childhood obesity, hypertension, high blood cholesterol and the emergence of maturity – onset type diabetes (Type 2 diabetes) in teenagers. <u>Maturity</u> onset diabetes (type 2 diabetes) used to be restricted to the <u>mature</u> person, but not these days. Generation Y now has Syndrome X and it is impacted by the X-Degeneration.

Many Americans may be ashamed to admit that we have the fattest kids in the world, with  evidence of the increasing emergence of the components of Syndrome X in our children. Furthermore, there is evidence of a steady decline in the level of aerobic fitness of children and teenagers. Where does this lead? Our pathway to ill health is determined largely by lifestyle. Whilst exercise, psychological well-being and the avoidance of substance abuse are pivotal for health, one must define nutrition as the simplest and potentially most effective approach to the eradication of chronic disease. This book reinforces the notion that nutritional change is especially relevant for impacting the killer constellation of problems found within Syndrome X.

The term "focus" of the intervention(s) as applied to prevent or treat heart disease is very important. In many respects, our "focus" on cardiovascular disease prevention has been "too focused". For example, the national preoccupation of treating high blood cholesterol alone, at the expense of correcting other cardiovascular risk factors (especially the other components of Syndrome X ) may be quite fallacious. Some evidence exists that there has been a phase of "prescription lunacy" in modern medicine, where cholesterol lowering drugs ( especially "statin" type drugs ) are prematurely applied to combat high blood cholesterol, without considering first line options such as diet, exercise and natural food supplements for lowering blood cholesterol. Whilst the terms, "prescription lunacy" seems harsh, there are many reasons not to overuse "statin – type" and other cholesterol-lowering drugs, especially in individuals without established cardiovascular disease or risks. Statin type drugs for lowering blood cholesterol have emerged with onerous adverse effects and questionable measures of cost and benefit.

Indeed, "statin type", cholesterol lowering drugs have recently been repeatedly associated with reports of side effects; and in one circumstance deaths have resulted in the removal of a  billion-dollar-selling, "statin" type of cholesterol-lowering medication. I believe that the "drug–focus" on blood cholesterol-lowering, which impacts only one aspect of many cardiovascular risk factors, may be replaced to a significant degree by remedies of natural origin or lifestyle interventions. "Natural interventions" are often able to address multiple risk factors simultaneously (all at the same time). In this book, I shall explain the versatile and potent ability of natural substances, such as special extracts of soluble fiber (beta glucans) and other dietary deletions or additions to combat Syndrome X.

No longer can some "hide-bound", allopathic physicians or conservative pharmaceutical companies deny the safety and effectiveness of many natural interventions to tackle the undesirable components of Syndrome X. Natural options such as beta glucan components of soluble fiber, may have more versatile effects than drugs and when used alone they may be able to combat more of the components of Syndrome X than many current drug treatments. Health Agencies of the Federal Government in the US have recently acknowledged the ability of natural supplements (or functional foods) to contribute to the prevention of disease, in particular the prevention of cardiovascular disease. Long delayed and eagerly anticipated US Government legislation to define "medical foods" is awaited. Striking examples of medical foods are components of soy and soluble fibers (beta-glucan fractions of oat soluble fiber) which carry tenable claims of health benefits, including an ability to balance blood glucose, lower cholesterol and, perhaps, assist in weight control.

The general public had been advised frequently to avoid the potential ineffectiveness of food or natural supplements as "medicine". However, nutritional scientists and many physicians have finally cemented their agreements on the overwhelming value of "food as medicine ". This circumstance is neither novel nor new. The dictum of "food is medicine" was proposed by Hippocrates, the father of modern medicine.

The information in this book is simplified by necessity, so that its messages can be within the reach of everyone, including our beloved youngsters. Healthcare-givers have grappled with the problems of changing behaviors towards a healthy lifestyle, but changing the dietary preferences of a nation is a monumental task. The good news is that "small" but positive corrections of adverse lifestyle can have major benefits on public health. This concept certainly applies in the lifestyle domain of nutrition. If only a small number people take a piece of advice on a healthy lifestyle change, when a common problem exists, then the health benefit can touch millions of people. My comments are not wishful thinking. Well conducted, scientific studies show the large scale health benefits of small, positive changes from "bad" to "good" lifestyle e.g. reduction in cigarette smoking, weight control, etc.

This book gives advice on both what individuals can do or what they can avoid to improve cardiovascular health by developing a specific combat plan against Syndrome X. It may tell a reader what they do not want to hear, especially when it comes to weight loss tactics. I deny the existence of a single diet for health and weight loss that suits everyone. Whilst the emphasis is on natural options, I do not reject the judicious application of drug or other conventional medical options. The medical approach in this book is pluralistic, but less emphasis is placed on conventional approaches, given the massive media advertising and overuse of drug therapy for disorders that have their basis primarily in disordered lifestyle.

I have referred to the ability of natural approaches to impact several cardiovascular risk factors in a simultaneous manner. A combined approach to reverse risks with lifestyle changes and natural interventions seems advantageous. Respected health promoting organizations such as the American Diabetes Association and the American Heart Association stress lifestyle issues as first line options. In the case of the American Diabetes Association, the drug treatment of maturity onset diabetes is referred to as the "back up plan", not the first line option. There are many clear examples of simple, versatile, safe and powerful health strategies to combat disease which utilize both common sense and remedies of natural origin.

If we take an example of a drug that lowers cholesterol and produces some measurable benefits against a background of cost and safety concerns, we can trigger a debate that opens a "can of worms". Compare the use of the "drug approach" with natural options that can lower cholesterol in an inexpensive and safe manner e.g. beta-glucan extracts of soluble fiber and partial dietary switches from animal to soy protein. Which approach represents the most attractive option? Clearly, the natural substances would be preferred, providing that they worked! Modern science has shown us that many "natural approaches" do work. An important focus of this book is to reveal the valuable and scientifically proven benefits of several natural, nutritional approaches to combat Syndrome X.

Convinced that we can prevent premature death and disability from cardiovascular disease, I propose lifestyle change and I attempt to further "plant" the idea of movement towards "plant-based" diets. This book does not call for a strict vegetarian lifestyle, but its message is more related to advice about "curbing" our "meat and fried potatoes" dietary habits. I make yet another call for a moderation of saturated fat and animal protein intake in the Standard American Diet (SAD). Whilst many call, few listen.

Safe and effective natural plant substances exist that can impact the multiple components of Syndrome X ( obesity, hypertension , high blood cholesterol and glucose intolerance or insulin resistance). The most striking example of a natural approach that I shall explain in this book is the secret of carefully prepared extracts of ubiquitous plant substances called soluble fibers (beta glucans). Whilst many people have heard about the use of dietary fiber for health, it is recent research that shows us just how powerful certain fractions of specific types of soluble fiber (beta glucans) may be in lowering blood cholesterol, balancing blood glucose and helping to promote weight loss. In other terms, these beta glucan fractions of soluble fiber can help reverse the cardinal features of the killer combination of disorders that comprise Syndrome X.

Why are we not using these natural or nutritional approaches to combat Syndrome X in a widespread manner? This question provokes explanations that are modern day contentions in medical practice. Our discovery process of new treatments (drugs) is often driven by a "for-profit" industry which feels a strong need to apply proprietary or patented products that can be sold at a premium price, preferably with economic exclusivity. Unfortunately, remedies of natural origin are not viewed as proprietary (or "patentable") by pharmaceutical ("drug") companies. I believe that this is an example of narrow thinking by the emperors of drug development. In my recent invited editorial in Pharmaventures, (Oxford, UK, 2001), I challenge the pharmaceutical industry to rethink some of their drug development strategies and point to the therapeutic power of certain components of remedies of natural origin, which, incidentally, can be patented.

Whilst one may not blame the pharmaceutical or biotechnology industry for their "tried and trusted", economically-rewarding approach, the incentive to develop and apply remedies of natural origin is insignificant in comparison with the use of drugs. Remedies of natural origin are not generally attractive options for "big business" that has to generate "big profits". Patients and physicians are inundated with "me-too" drugs. In fact, billions of dollars are spent on creating similar drugs to do the same thing e.g. lower cholesterol, treat arthritis etc. In contrast, only a relative "pittance" exists in research money to develop dietary supplements, remedies of natural origin and many beneficial functional food components.

I have emphasized the "secret of soluble fiber" in this book, because I believe that the use of selected extracts of fiber (beta glucans) can fundamentally change the health of our nation in a low cost, effective and safe manner. The "secret of soluble fiber" is not really a secret, it explains the physical and chemical characteristics of certain types of fiber that have both "physical" actions and intrinsic metabolic effects (IMEF), i.e. they change body chemistry. I have been a protagonist of soy protein and fish oil for the promotion of cardiovascular health in two of my previous books "The Soy Revolution" (Dell Publishing, NY, NY, 2000) and "The Natural Way to a Healthy Heart" (M. Evans Publishing, NY, NY, 1999). Some of the discussions in this book on soluble fiber relate primarily to extensions to my own published research in the journal "Lancet", in 1979. My colleagues and I performed some of the early studies the beneficial effect of soluble fibers on glucose (sugar) absorption in humans. I shall explain how, this work formed part of the physiological basis of what nutritionists now call the "glycemic index" of foods.

Earlier observations of my colleagues and I on the mechanism of action of plant soluble fibers on gastrointestinal function have been complemented by highly complex agricultural, biochemical, nutritional and basic science experiments performed in the early 1990's. These studies revealed the "hidden", beneficial properties of soluble fiber. Previously, dietary fiber had often been considered to be a relatively "inert" dietary ingredient. Quite to the contrary, its complex chemistry and physical nature make it a powerful substrate in our diet. I reiterate that there is an intrinsic metabolic effect (IMEF) of soluble fiber that can help explain its role in cholesterol lowering, colon health and appetite control. I am not minimizing the value of other natural plant substances (herbals or botanicals) that can play a major role in promoting cardiovascular health. Nor am I rejecting appropriate allopathic (drug) therapies. My approach in this book is "pluralistic."

Many contemporary scientists share my viewpoint on the unhealthy nature of our Standard American Diet (SAD). I am convinced that the Western diet is too high in the wrong types of carbohydrates and poorly selected meat and dairy products. However, many people respond to the "meat and dairy lobby" which wishes to acknowledge and amplify some of the general nutritional values of these apparent "nourishing traditions". Meat comes often with an excessive load of saturated fat and cholesterol, as may standard milk products. In this book, I reveal how a small move in our diet towards vegetable-sources of protein and complex carbohydrates can make a big difference to the "bouquet of barbed wire" of risk factors that cause cardiovascular disease (particularly the components of Syndrome X). There is, however, a healthy way of utilizing or modifying standard meat and milk products to make them healthier. I describe how modern food technology permits the incorporation of soluble fiber into milk that provides the option of a new "healthful" type of milk drink. Additions of specific types of soluble fiber can impact cholesterol, or "sugar" problems (diabetes) and weight control. This new use of food or beverages as medicine has been variably termed the development of "functional beverages" or "functional foods". In the case of beverages, certain functional foods components (e.g. beta glucans) can be added to drinks so that they have a positive, far-reaching, health function.

Unfortunately, it is difficult to motivate "young" people to make lifestyle or specific nutritional changes that represent an investment for future health. The gustatory delights of high saturated fat intake are a powerful reinforcement to continue adverse dietary behavior, especially when the idea of future health is remote; even though it is important. In this book, I present some natural options that are within the reach of many people (including children) to impact the combination of risk factors within Syndrome X. Furthermore, I emphasize that it is never too late to derive a benefit from positive nutritional or lifestyle changes. Furthermore, I am

confident that the mature individual and the elderly will benefit
from the advice given in this book.

Accepting that the eradication of heart disease could extend
our natural life expectancy by twenty years, many more Americans
would be pushing a 100 years of age with significant reductions in
cardiovascular risks and, in turn, heart disease. Humankind lives
with a misconception, fostered somewhat by the "worshippers of
high technology", that there is a new "drug" or a treatment on the
horizon that may solve all of our illnesses. Not only have we "never
been so wrong" in terms of an expectation, the death and disability rate from obesity, high blood cholesterol and cardiovascular
disease is stubbornly high and rising in some specific circumstances.
A strong argument exists that the recently-recorded, small, decline
in deaths from heart disease, observed in recent years, has little to
do with drugs, surgery or "high- tech" medicine. I believe that this
positive trend  in a reduction of cardiovascular deaths has more to
do with a change of lifestyle. This book stresses these latter options,
but I have not turned my back on the credible and important
advances in modern medicine that can combat disease e.g. the
expert, emergency management of a heart attack.

If a person has a need for a drug or surgery (allopathic medicines) they must exercise the correct option, especially in the presence of a medical emergency. In most circumstances, lowering blood
cholesterol, engaging in weight control and balancing modest
changes in blood glucose are not medical emergencies. Again, I
stress the "first–line–approach" must consider the safe and gentle
options which often involve a lifestyle adjustment, particularly a
nutritional or dietary change. The "stroke" of the prescription the
pen and the "flash" of the surgeon's knife are not perceived to be
as attractive to patients as they once were. Although natural
approaches to disease prevention make economic, political and
social sense, they have been rejected somewhat over the past fifty
years, especially in the name of some allopathic (conventional) medical advances. Some of these "advances" have been of dubious value
and, overall, they exert relatively little impact on reducing the occurrence of (preventing) cardiovascular and other diseases. Natural
approaches to disease prevention and treatment have more power
and versatility than hitherto supposed.

During the writing of this book, I found much of the scientific information on the importance of insulin resistance in the genesis of Syndrome X to be complex and in some circumstances incomplete. Whilst insulin resistance links many of the components of Syndrome X, other factors operate. Therefore, I ran the danger of presenting too many complex scientific arguments to support the validity of certain conclusions. I admit that a general consensus does not exist on every component of my reasoning on how to combat Syndrome X, but I have attempted to separate speculation from fact. I am not brokering conventional or alternative medicine, but I am looking for what works in a cost-effective, simple, safe and effective manner by applying the principles of "medical pluralism". I stress, however, that this book does not provide a comprehensive review of conventional, medical options for Syndrome X and cardiovascular disease. The primary reason for my approach is to seek alternatives, given the success of conventional medicine in some areas and its predictable failure in others.

I trust that this book will not be perceived as "just" another book about how to "just" lower blood cholesterol or "just" get thin etc. Its message is much broader and if not recognized as such, its impact will be lost. This work is written for everyone in the hope that it will inform the layperson and not induce somnolence in the healthcare professional. It weaves natural and conventional medicine together in the quest for cardiovascular health. I admit some distaste for terms such as alternative medicine, conventional medicine and complementary medicine. As we enter the new millennium, medical advances lie at the interface of healthcare disciplines. This circumstance dictates a requirement for caregivers to think "pluralistically" and adopt an integrated medical approach. Indeed, the age of "pluralistic" medicine is upon us.

During my work as a member of a health task force, appointed by the Institute of Medicine (Washington DC), in the late 1980's, I witnessed the acceptance by the US Government of recommendations for lifestyle adjustments as a key to health. This focus on positive lifestyle change for health was embraced with unanimity among the assembled health experts. Although the conclusions of the Task Force were accepted by the US Government, they were not completely enacted. In fact, many may have been ignored. Nothing about the concept of disease prevention by lifestyle adjustment was new at that stage. Why should it be per-

ceived as debatable as we move into a new millennium? Innovative
scientists, politicians, and physicians have pointed convincingly at
the benefit of correcting adverse lifestyle, especially nutrition, for
one hundred years or more. Unfortunately, "lifestyle plans" are
still not part of mainstream healthcare, even though they are touted
by "managed care"..

    This book is part of my ambition to motivate some health-
care-givers and the general public to endorse several obvious, natural but overlooked solutions to cardiovascular wellness. If some
of my writings sound "like a broken record", I stress that this
approach is intentional, in order to "hammer home lessons" that
we have not learned. I have attempted to do this by presenting facts
and describing the interrelationship among the constellation of
problems that form Syndrome X. Syndrome X or Syndrome X, Y
and Z... encompass the intertwined risks of cardiovascular disability and death within "the bouquet of barbed wire". My hypothesis within the domains of "combat Syndrome X" marries
conventional medicine with several valid but underestimated natural options for cardiovascular health. Please read this book with
optimism. I hope that some healthcare givers and patients will gain
a different perspective on the use of "combined" approaches involving allopathic medicine and nutrition to tackle humankind's number one enemy, namely Syndrome X, Y and Z... and its ensuing
diseases.

    Stephen Holt, M.D., January 2002

# HOW TO USE THIS BOOK

The causes and outcomes of Syndrome X or Syndrome X, Y and Z... are not fully understood. My book involves a discussion of some concepts that are readily understood, but it does contain overviews of scientific material that may be not readily comprehended by the individual without formal biomedical training. For this reason, the book has both standard sized text and small print. The standard, font size is for everyone to read but the smaller print may be only fully understood by individuals with more advanced scientific knowledge. I have tried to make the book more universally appealing by adopting this approach, but I cannot expect my messages to come across by baffling the lay person or boring the "scientist". I acknowledge that attempts to please everyone are usually unsuccessful or impossible.

**Questions?** Write e-mail to info@combatsyndromex.com

# SPECIAL NOTE TO READERS

"Combat Syndrome X, Y and Z..." reflects the author's opinion of how to impact risk factors that cause or contribute to cardiovascular and other diseases. It represents the authors interpretation of scientific, medical and popular literature. The book is not intended to interfere with the valuable doctor-client relationship and it is not a substitute for medical consultation or appropriate treatment or advice on disease prevention from a healthcare professional. Quite to the contrary, the author recommends that you share the viewpoints in this book with healthcare professionals and he does not recommend self- medication in the presence of significant illness. In any cases of doubt, the author and publisher recommend that readers seek medical advice. The book is not intended to promote or sell a specific product and the publisher or author accepts no responsibility for the use of any substances mentioned in this book. Syndrome X or Syndrome X, Y and Z... form a serious constellation of disorders with serious consequences. The author believes that his interpretations of natural approaches will help combat Syndrome X, Y and Z... in a highly positive manner.

# SYNDROME X: THE KILLER COMBINATION

## THE EPIDEMIC OF SYNDROME X

Obesity, high blood cholesterol and blood pressure, with the pivotal underlying state of insulin resistance, constitute Syndrome X (Figure 1). This Syndrome affects seventy million (or more) Americans, but most of these victims are unaware of its presence. Given increasing awareness of this disorder among healthcare givers, many people are waiting to be told that they have this potentially fatal disorder. Recent literature has characterized Syndrome X as the "silent killer" or the "unknown epidemic", making it deserving of the label "X" and identifying it as a disorder worthy of the formation of a battle plan for "combat". At the annual meeting of the American Heart Association in 2001 the terms Syndrome X were "buzz words".

Syndrome X was christened more than ten years ago, but its discovery goes back to 1965, or thereabouts, and it is based on the many years of work of Dr. Gerald Reaven MD, of Stanford University, California and others. Like many significant medical discoveries that are somewhat contrarian to prevailing medical opinion, Dr. Reaven's enlightened research on Syndrome X was initially ignored. Early responses from the medical community to the proposals of Dr. Reaven, and his colleagues, on the importance of the body's resistance to signals from insulin were "frosty". Even these days, some physicians and scientists claim that Syndrome X may not even exist!

Despite some prevailing rhetoric, many medical researchers are working hard to uncover the disorders of body chemistry that cause Syndrome X and, predictably, the pharmaceutical industry is looking for "drugs" that balance blood sugar, by overcoming insulin resistance and lower cholesterol. This new drug development strategy is relying heavily on "unzipping" the human genome in the practice of pharmaceutical biotechnology. Whilst there are some insulin-sensitizing drugs available, the first of these drugs was withdrawn because of liver toxicity and deaths; and these types of medication may on occasion cause a rise in blood cholesterol and body weight. In anticipation of new drug discoveries for Syndrome X, advertising sponsored by the pharmaceutical industry is "educating" physicians and potential patients on the nature of Syndrome X. In this book, you will discover the interplay of the disorders within Syndrome X and learn about the existence of reliable, "natural" options to overcome the constellation of problems within Syndrome X, which may be extended to the concept of Syndrome X, Y and Z...

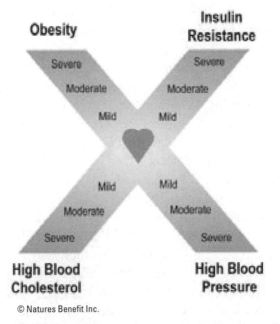

© Natures Benefit Inc.

**Figure 1:** The multidimensional components of Syndrome X which account for cardiovascular risks. Note: Each component can be variably present and the manifestations of this disorder are protean.

# The Typical X–MAN or X–WOMAN?

Whilst proclaiming the occurrence of a new disease or syndrome, a clear recognition of the new entity is demanded by the listeners. No such luck, when it comes to the availability of clear descriptions of Syndrome X! In its classic presentation, it occurs in a mature man or woman who is obese ("apple shaped"), suffering from high blood pressure and cholesterol with insulin resistance or pre–type 2 diabetes mellitus. In some forms of Syndrome X, these disorders are variably present making many indistinct boundaries among the combination of disorders within Syndrome X (Figure 1). There are other manifestations of Syndrome X that are even more "hidden". Young women with Syndrome X can present with irregular menstruation, obesity, acne, excessive body hair, polycystic ovaries and infertility. There is mounting evidence that disorders of male reproductive function are often caused by Syndrome X and Syndrome X in pregnancy presents itself as "Gestational Diabetes". Syndrome X compounds health risks for mature women and men "going through" the menopause or andropause, respectively. This makes the recognition of this syndrome difficult in many cases and it reinforces my license to use the new concepts of Syndrome X, Y and Z....

Within the complex of disorders comprising Syndrome X, about one in ten (10%), or more, of individuals develop diabetes mellitus with overt evidence of uncontrolled blood sugar. Furthermore, to fall into the diagnostic category of Syndrome X, people do not necessarily have to be fat or have high blood pressure (hypertension). Dr. Reaven has proposed that there is a metabolic defect (altered body chemistry) that causes resistance to insulin. This metabolic defect is caused by a combination of hereditary and lifestyle factors. In other words, insulin is present but it does not do its job properly. It is the resistance to insulin that sets the stage for obesity, high blood cholesterol and hypertension. These days, many scientists are trying to unravel the disordered body chemistry that accounts for Syndrome X and some are convinced that it has a hereditary (genetic) basis (at least in part) with one or more genes accounting for the disorder. Whatever the genetic basis of Syndrome X, environmental issues play a major role in shaping Syndrome X.

To date, there is no unifying theory for the cause of Syndrome X, even though many medical detectives are convinced that altered responses to insulin trigger many aspects of Syndrome X. Several components of Syndrome X, including glucose intolerance due to insulin resistance (pre–diabetes mellitus) and hypertension, are more common among Native Americans, Mexican Americans and female African Americans. Dr. Gerald Reaven and his colleagues indicated, with clarity, that non-Caucasians in the US are at greater risk for Syndrome X, but current trends are for an alarming increase in the occurrence of this disorder in all ethnic groups, in many "developed" nations.

## US Adults with Syndrome X

In January 2002, US Federal Government researchers examined records collected on approximately 9000 men and women over the age of 20 years between 1988 and 1994, to provide an indirect estimate the occurrence of Syndrome X (the metabolic syndrome) in the population (Ford ES, Giles WH, Dietz W, JAMA, 297, 3, 356-359, 2002). According to these researchers, who adopted an incomplete definition of Syndrome X, it was found that approximately 47 million adults in the US had the disorder. This information was collected almost a decade ago and it is likely to be currently an underestimate of the problem.

The information collected by the researchers was considered to have serious socioeconomic consequences for the US. Referring to the unrelenting epidemic of obesity, inappropriate nutritional practices and lack of exercise facing Americans, there was a call for comprehensive efforts to combat the metabolic Syndrome X.

The researchers provided a definition of Syndrome X (the metabolic syndrome) in the following manner:

-   Abdominal obesity: waist circumference greater than 102 cm in men and greater than 88 cm in women;
-   Hypertriglyceridemia: greater than 150 mg/dL (1.69 mmol/I);
-   Low high-density lipoprotein (HDL) cholesterol: less than 40 mg/dL (1.04 mmol/L) in men and less than 50 mg/dL (1.29 mmol/L) in women;

- High blood pressure: greater than 140/85 mm Hg;
- High fasting glucose: greater than 110 mg/dL ( 6.1 mmol/L).

I believe that the above definition of Syndrome X, used in the third report of the National Cholesterol Education Expert Panel (on detection evaluation and treatment of high blood cholesterol), requires revision and a more complete and validated definition of Syndrome X and diagnostic indices are required (see Section 10, The Syndrome X Clinical Index). The recent reports of the emergence of Syndrome X stress cardiovascular disease morbidity (illness) and mortality (deaths) but they tend to downplay the other consequences of this disorder (e.g. polycystic ovary syndrome, infertility, liver disease, cancer) which increase illness and death from many other causes (the concept of Syndrome X, Y and Z...).

There seems to be a reluctance among some medical practitioners, including the Federal Government research teams, to use the term Syndrome X and there is a tendency to refer to Syndrome X as "the metabolic syndrome" . To label a disorder "metabolic syndrome" without knowing completely the derangements of "metabolism" within "Syndrome X" has created problems. Perhaps the suggestion that we think in broader terms such as Syndrome X, Y and Z... serves a useful purpose? There may be a "meeting of minds" when the Federal Government researchers state "...it seems unlikely that management of the individual abnormalities of this syndrome provides better outcomes than a more integrated strategy" (JAMA, 3, 297, p. 359, 2002). An integrated strategy is the precise direction that I propose in this book, with much bias towards the prevention of Syndrome X.

## UNDERSTANDING THE GENESIS OF SYNDROME X

Throughout this book, I shall emphasize (and reiterate) the multidimensional causes of cardiovascular disease. Syndrome X is, in itself, a collection of both diseases and risk disorders. Understanding how the disorders fit together in Syndrome X, to cause risks for cardiovascular disease, requires an understanding of the actions of insulin which are sometimes recognized in an incomplete manner. Some of the less obvious actions of insulin are unfamiliar to the general public and some healthcare givers.

Insulin is a hormone secreted by cells within the pancreas gland (located in the abdomen, behind the stomach) and it coordinates certain cells (tissues) of the body to take up glucose by assimilating this sugar from the bloodstream. Thus, insulin feeds cells with sugar (fuel). Without insulin, blood sugar levels in the blood become high and other serious changes in body chemistry can occur. This is essentially what occurs in a type of diabetes where insulin lack is the hallmark. This type of diabetes is called Type 1 diabetes (Juvenile Onset Diabetes), but Type 1 diabetes is less relevant to understanding Syndrome X than is Type 2 diabetes (Maturity Onset Diabetes).

In Syndrome X (and in some early forms of Type 2 diabetes mellitus, prediabetes), the body may produce a lot of insulin (hyperinsulinism). This overproduction of insulin occurs because the cells of the body do not take instructions from the hormone insulin and the pancreas responds by secreting "too much" insulin. In other words, the body develops a resistance to the commands from insulin to control blood sugar. This is what is commonly referred to as insulin resistance.

It is the resistance to insulin, or failure of the body to act on insulins' instructions that triggers Syndrome X. This trigger is not simple. It results in a whole series of events which damage body tissues and change body functions. Blood vessels of the cardiovascular system are a particular focus of damage and protein metabolism changes in the body. Excess insulin switches body chemistry towards the production of chemicals that promote inflammation (change in eicosanoid status) and excess insulin can help switch on certain genes that are involved in cancer. Excessive insulin circulates in the blood in many cases of Syndrome X and it can result in less well known effects of insulin that become magnified in their effects. This type of insulin excess causes the liver to manufacture cholesterol and load the blood with fats (high blood cholesterol and triglycerides); and it encourages the body to store more fat, thereby promoting obesity. Increases in fats in the blood ("bad cholesterol") causes deposition of fat in arterial blood vessels and clogs them. This deposition of fat is called atheroma. Atheroma leads to poor circulation, stroke, angina and heart attack or coronary heart disease.

It is clear that the description of Syndrome X includes many of the known risk factors of heart disease or stroke, e.g. high blood cholesterol, hypertension etc. All of the derangements in body structure and function found in Syndrome X spell great trouble for cardiovascular health. Overall, this circumstance is especially relevant to the occurrence of high blood cholesterol where the stimulus of excessive insulin can push blood fats to levels that dramatically increase a persons' risks of heart attack, stroke and coronary heart disease.

## A GROWING EPIDEMIC

As Syndrome X occurs more frequently or is diagnosed more often, individuals with this disorder are often "loaded-up" with prescription drugs that address the separate components of the syndrome. Discussions of this type of polypharmacy (multiple drug therapy) have reached the financial press in recent times. An article in Forbes Magazine (August, 6, 2001) by Mary Ellen Egan describes the polypharmacy (multiple drug therapy) in some individuals with Syndrome X. She describes the unfortunate circumstance of an individual with Syndrome X on an anti-hypertensive drug combined with two anti-diabetic drugs and a cholesterol lowering drug at a monthly cost of US$ 485. Whilst safety and efficacy of drug treatments require great debate, the costs of drug therapy used to address the components of Syndrome X are staggering.

The epidemic of Syndrome X is growing and the use of drugs to combat this disorder is also growing. These trends are alarming when one just accounts for the "health cost" of the side effects of drugs used to treat the components of Syndrome X. In later chapters of this book, I shall explore how natural options exist to combat Syndrome X, without applying an "exclusively-drug-approach". I shall emphasize how drug treatment is sometimes of dubious benefit. Whilst several drug companies are working on drugs that can assist the body to process sugar and fats, thereby helping to regulate blood glucose and cholesterol together, there is a long way to go in this pathway of drug development. We cannot wait five or more years for drug makers to find versatile pharmaceuticals that impact the spectrum of problems within Syndrome X.

Early attempts to discover drugs to combat insulin resistance (Syndrome X) have been variably successful, with an example of one new, partially-effective drug (troglitazone) being removed from the market. This drug caused severe liver problems and occasional deaths. Less well known was the fact that this drug may have had limited effects on overcoming insulin resistance at the expense of causing a rise in blood cholesterol in some cases. These recent experiences are not pharmaceutical triumphs, they are "iatrogenic-disease-disasters". Pharmaceutical companies have begun educational programs for both physicians and consumers on Syndrome X, in anticipation of the development of new drugs. However, this educational process is not focused on the "here and now" and it is not likely to be extended to extol any virtues of viable preventive or treatment options with natural food supplements or functional foods.

## BREEDING SYNDROME X

In this book, I hope to motivate people who are variably overweight, glucose intolerant, hypertensive and hypercholesterolemic to recognize this killer combination of problems and take positive steps to combat their ownership of the "metabolic", Syndrome X. Perhaps we are "fed up" with being told that we are getting fatter, less fit and dying prematurely of cardiovascular disease. Indeed, we have justifiable reasons to feel "fed up" and even scared. The reality is that there is an epidemic of obesity, hypertension, high blood cholesterol and insulin resistance which has been defined somewhat "loosely" under the term Syndrome X, but it is amenable to correction.

Despite billions of dollars being spent on weight control tactics and drug treatments for diabetic and cardiovascular ailments, our death rate from the combination of insulin resistance, glucose intolerance and heart or circulatory disease remains shockingly high (see Section 10). I wish to reiterate that Syndrome X has the variable presence of obesity, abnormal blood fats (lipids, cholesterol), degrees of insulin resistance ( pre – diabetic or diabetic states) and high blood pressure(Figure 1). Whilst a "syndrome" is defined as a collection of symptoms and signs, indicative of a disease, Syndrome X has variable manifestations and it does not breed true in its presentation. It is a "mongrel" disorder which requires repeated reappraisal as we attempt to eliminate its causes.

The components of Syndrome X threaten every adult and many teenagers in Western nations. I believe the term Syndrome X (coined by Gerald Reaven MD) is very valuable because it emphasizes the interplay of a combination of disorders that determine our primary cause of death and disability, notably cardiovascular disease. Whilst the label Syndrome X is valuable, it has limitations as we explore the significance of this disorder to other diseases such as female infertility, acne, cystic ovaries, immune impairments, cancer and chronic inflammation (the concept of "Syndrome X, Y and Z..."). Despite prevailing contentions, the constellation (combination) of problems encountered in Syndrome X seem to fit together in an incomplete, "jig saw" puzzle that explains the genesis of the number one killer in society – cardiovascular (CVS) disease.

## ADVERSE LIFESTYLE PROMOTES DISEASE.

It is matter of fact that many people are doing many things wrong in terms of their lifestyle. The question remains: Beyond simple advice, what can we do to reverse these undesirable circumstances? The answer rests in public education and an understanding of the lifestyle factors that contribute to the different disorders described within Syndrome X (Table 1). "Adverse lifestyles" are readily defined by behavioral scientists and those domains (areas) of lifestyle that predispose to the modern epidemic of Syndrome X can be described in new terms as "The X Factors" (Table 2). Understanding these "X factors" (Table 2) will permit a rational approach to combat their nefarious influence on the health of our society.

| Factor | Significance |
|---|---|
| Diet | A high saturated fat content of diet may potentiate coronary artery disease. Saturated fat is bad, essential fatty acids e.g. fish oil are good. Simple sugars are readily converted to body fat. |
| Blood Lipids (*) | Risk of atheroma is directly proportionate to the increase in concentration of total cholesterol and of low density lipoprotein (LDL) and |

inversely proportionate to concentration of high density lipoprotein (HDL). High triglycerides (a hallmark of Syndrome X) is a major risk.

Blood Pressure (*)    Risk is directly proportionate to the increase of systolic or diastolic blood pressure.

Cigarette Smoking    Risk is proportionate to the number of cigrettes smoked per day (risk is 3 times control at a pack or more of cigarettes per day).

Personality Type    A competitive, driving person (so-called Type A personality) is more prone to coronary artery disease. The aggressive, conversation-interrupting male is a great risk.

Sedentary Living    Individuals who do not exercise regularly may have a greater risk of myocardial infarction than do individuals who exercise regularly.

Diabetes Mellitus (*)    Risk is 2 times control in diabetic men, 3 times control in diabetic women. (the issue of insulin resistance, without established diabetes, as a risk factor is of paramount importance).

Obesity (*)    Fat people have more coronary artery disease than those of normal body habitus.

**Table 1: Risk Factors for Coronary Artery and other Diseases:**
Although alcohol and caffeine have been claimed by some to be independent risk factors, they have not been established to be clear risks. However, obesity, by increasing the severity of hypertension, hyperlipidemia, and diabetes mellitus, may have an important influence on the development of coronary artery disease. This is the basis of Syndrome X. The four cardinal components of the metabolic Syndrome X, Y and Z .... are denoted by an asterisk (*).

## THE X FACTORS

The recognition of Syndrome X (Figure 1) and its importance as a cause of cardiovascular disease and deaths must make us rethink the "classic" list of cardiovascular risk factors (Table 1). Figure 1 shows the combination of disorders within Syndrome X and it is depicted in a multidimensional manner. One must address the X factors (Table 2), that compound cardiovascular risks in order to understand the ways to combat Syndrome X.

- Insulin resistance
- Obesity
- High blood insulin levels
- High blood "bad" cholesterol (LDL)
- High blood triglycerides
- Low blood "good" cholesterol (HDL)
- Slow clearance of fats from blood
- Stimuli to cholesterol synthesis in the liver
- Tendency to blood clotting
- Adverse lifestyle e.g. smoking, lack of exercise etc.
    which aggravates insulin resistance
- High blood uric acid
- High blood homocysteine levels*

**Table 2:** The X-factors: A novel list of risk factors for cardiovascular (CVS) disease incorporating more of the risk factors within Syndrome X. This list is based on concepts proposed by several scientists. I have added elevated blood homocysteine to the X factors because of its link to cardiovascular disease, perhaps by the "wasting" of B vitamins that occurs with hyperglycemia.

The X factors should be added to standard cardiovascular risk factors to expand the definition of currently acknowledged cardiovascular risks; and, as such, their identification cannot be considered novel or new. Among these X factors (Table 2) are many aspects of the four cardinal components of Syndrome X that were highlighted in Table 1 and Figure 1 (obesity, hypertension, high blood cholesterol and insulin resistance). Modern medicine has clung to rigid definitions of cardiovascular risk (Table 1) by only highlighting a risk factor if it can be shown to operate in an independent manner. This research has contributed to a treatment approach to cardiovascular disease that has been too focused on dealing with one risk factor, e.g. lowering blood cholesterol or controlling blood pressure with drugs at the expense of global combat against all risks.

Appeasement of the dictated burden of scientific proof to show one or other factor operating as an independent risk for cardiovascular disease has tended to prevent a more global approach to combat cardiovascular disease. Furthermore, medical advances that can be applied to combat Syndrome X have been hampered in their application by focused research on individual cardiovascular risk factors, e.g. "just" lowering cholesterol. "Just" lowering cholesterol with a drug results in the correction of only one risk factor, but this approach may not combat cardiovascular disease with any efficiency (lack of cost-effectiveness and occurrence onerous drug side effects). Table 2 expands our knowledge of cardiovascular risk by looking at cardiovascular risk components of Syndrome X, Y and Z.... in greater detail. (the X-factors)

## Parts of a Bigger Jig–Saw Puzzle of Cardiovascular Risk

I reiterate that one of the best examples of "focused" research in cardiovascular disease is the preoccupation with lowering blood cholesterol with drugs (see Section 2). Whilst elevated blood cholesterol is undoubtedly important in the causation of cardiovascular disease, it is not the whole story. High blood cholesterol is certainly an example of an important component of our revised list of cardiovascular risks that highlights the X factors (Table 2). Correcting elevated blood cholesterol is only a few pieces of the bigger jig-saw puzzle which fits together in terms of Syndrome X and cardiovascular risks (Table 2) or Syndrome X, Y and Z....

To attempt to define Syndrome X with clarity is important. Figure 1 starts to define the complex nature of Syndrome X and the factors that operate within Syndrome X are listed in Table 2. We recognize Syndrome X as a variable mixture of disordered blood lipids, high blood pressure, abnormalities of blood glucose regulation, often combined with obesity. The key issue is to recognize that each factor (disorder or condition) may operate to a variable degree and produce variants within the frame-work of Syndrome X. For example, obesity may predominate or high blood cholesterol can dominate the overall picture of Syndrome X. Regardless of the combination of the variables, the end result is an excessive cardiovascular risk, with the ultimate occurrence of disabilities of several types and a tendency to premature death (the concept of Syndrome X, Y and Z...). Thus, the combined cardiovascular risks that we must consider include classic risks (Table 1) with added risks shown in Table 2. The "X factors" in Table 2 form a bigger jig saw puzzle of cardiovascular risk, but the identity of the "finished jig saw puzzle" is still somewhat indistinct.

## CARDIOVASCULAR RISK FACTORS: INEXTRICABLE LINKAGE

Elevated blood cholesterol is one major factor that is inextricably linked to other cardiovascular disease risk factors. It is a key component of Syndrome X. However, I reiterate that many other risk factors aggregate together to promote heart attack, coronary heart disease and stroke. Medical research has shown that stress, obesity, cigarette smoking and genetic predispositions are often linked to high blood cholesterol and the risk of coronary heart disease (Table 1). These factors operate together in compounding the risk of heart attack and ischemic heart disease (starvation of blood to the heart muscle). The greater the number of risk factors present the greater the risks. One must again reflect that coronary heart disease remains the number one killer in Western Society.

## "KILLING YOU SOFTLY"

Cardiovascular risks that are illustrated in Table 1 and the components of Syndrome X (Figure 1 and Table 2) compound themselves as a health threat. Thus, the X factors (Table 2) are "Killing You Softly" often over an extended period of time. It has been often overlooked that components of Syndrome X,(including high blood cholesterol obesity, hypertension and glucose intolerance) affect our children increasingly and heart disease may start in a silent manner in children and teenagers. Substance abuse is very important in compounding risks and initiating some of the components of Syndrome X. In particular, the risks of cigarette smoking and excessive alcohol intake are directly related to quantity, frequency and duration of consumption. The earlier the lifestyle (or nutritional) intervention to correct cardiovascular risk factors (or to prevent any component of Syndrome X), the better the prognosis (outcome). Impacting risk factors early in life will save lives and promote health in our loved ones.

## The "Bouquet of Barbed Wire"

Recent scientific research continues to provide evidence of close linkage among cardiovascular disease risk factors. The concept of Syndrome X has its power in recognizing the interconnections of the disorders and the compounded risks for cardiovascular disease. Many studies show that hypercholesterolemia (high blood cholesterol) goes hand in hand with stress, smoking and obesity. Obesity is linked with hypertension and sedentary occupations. Lack of physical activity causes obesity, especially in children. Smoking causes heart disease and may precipitate heart attack. The permutation of associations of health risk factors are variable and often complex (Tables 1 and 2). This is the "bouquet of barbed wire" that tightens around many people and it may be "Killing You Softly".

## Adverse Lifestyle is a Key Silent Killer

The common thread of thought that aids in the understanding of the causes of coronary artery disease is the recognition that the overall risk is most often related to adverse lifestyle (see Section 6, Lifestyle to Combat Syndrome X). There is no doubt that poor nutrition figures strongly in the risks. Adverse lifestyle creates domains of "risk behavior" that form the complex "bouquet of barbed wire" of risk factors. I stress that the "bouquet of barbed wire" chokes life and kills with silence. Whilst most individuals can spot if they are too fat, smoke too much or engage in risky behavior, many individuals continue to maintain their risks in an unimpeded manner. We have learned that multiple cardiovascular risk factors add up to potentially more serious cardiovascular risks and consequences. Furthermore, it is recognized that the dangers of coronary heart disease and heart attack increase as the number of risk factors increase. The famous Framingham Heart

Study, which is often quoted in medical circles, taught us about the additive nature of cardiovascular risk factors. The recognition and correction of these risk factors is at the "heart" of prevention programs, proposed by the American Heart Association and other leading bodies of opinion.

## How to succumb to the "Killing You Softly"

Many popular health books stress changes that are necessary to promote well-being. This approach may not be quite as effective as pointing out the ways to ensure ill health (Table 3).

| Lifestyle Approach to Poor Health | Comments |
|---|---|
| Smoke Heavily | Safe levels of smoking defy clear definition. |
| Drink Alcohol Excessively | If you do not die of liver disease you will succumb to trauma usually after very painful social isolation. |
| Stay Fat | Significant obesity is clearly associated with chronic disease and early death. |
| Do Not Exercise | This assures many health problems and a lack of well-being. |
| Stress Yourself Constantly | You may become distraught, mentally or physically ill and persecute others. |
| Eat a Lousy Diet | Good way to make almost every organ in the body fail. |
| Ignore Conventional Medical Practitioners | He or she could save your life. |
| Ignore Nutritionally Orientated Physicians | He or she has a lot to offer and can enhance the quality of your life. |

| | |
|---|---|
| Do Not Have Periodic Health Checks | You will never know much about your risks of illness or death. You will die in ignorance. |
| Self-Medicate With Pharmaceuticals | Over-the-counter medications are freely available for you to abuse and some are lethal when misused. |
| Take Excessive Quantities of "Health Foods", Dietary Supplements or "way-out" Herbal Cures | You can ruin your health with excessive vitamin intake. Many dietary supplements have "purposely" misleading health claims. Some herbs are great poisons. |
| Make Your Own Diagnosis and Ignore Prolonged or Serious Symptoms | There are many serious diseases that can kill you slowly. Several are amenable to cure. Self- medication or diagnosisis is a great way of denying yourself a good health outcome. |
| Engage in Risk Lifestyles | It may be pleasurable to put your life at risk and it is easy to die prematurely. |

**Table 3:** Some sure tactics for poor health. NOTE: These are not recommendations for anyone to follow. They are written and expressed in a manner that is designed to stimulate thoughts about lifestyle change that could accrue to an individual's benefit.

## THE PLEASURE OF ADVERSE LIFESTYLE

Adverse lifestyle is pleasurable for many and it is often subject to convenient thinking (mental dynamisms) such as denial, projection or rationalization (see Section 6 on lifestyle): "Mental dynamisms" were described by the Viennese psychiatrist Sigmund Freud who was once considered to be a pervert by his colleagues and many members of European society. There is a large body of scientific evidence to support the notion that most people minimize their indulgence in adverse lifestyles. The person who has an "over-eating disorder" at the root of his or her problem of obesity is highly likely to underestimate the quantity and quality of food that they consume on a daily basis. Fast food has become a staple diet for many, but it is often loaded with unhealthy types of saturated fat, simple sugars and cholesterol. It is a normal human reaction to suppress the significance of a health risk, especially if maintaining the risk is pleasurable. Who doesn't like burgers, twinkies, pies and fries?

Many other factors reinforce the perpetuation of adverse lifestyle. Excessive drinking, overeating and smoking have powerful social endorsement. Excess intake of the wrong type of dietary fat is a major factor in the causation of coronary heart disease, but fat tastes good to many. Even some "diet gurus" have misinformed society that saturated fat intake is a healthy way to lose weight! Furthermore, many people have acted on the misinformation. Scientific studies show that excessive dietary fat intake (especially saturated fat) is closely related to the development of obesity, overeating, cardiovascular disease and cancer. To believe in the high, unhealthy fat diet, disguised as the sometimes, meritorious, "low carb" lifestyle is a common mistake. On the one hand, high saturated fat diets and high protein diets have begun to masquerade under the label "low carb lifestyle", whereas on the other hand, the "low fat lifestyle" may disguise high "simple" sugar diets (see Section 5, Obesity and the Slim Chance).

| Popular Fast Food Items | Grams of Fat Per Average Serving: |
|---|---|
| Whopper Burger | 36 |
| Burrito Supreme | 22 |
| Deluxe Hamburger | 21 |
| Sausage Biscuit with Egg | 33 |
| Popcorn Chicken | 45 |
| Quarter Pounder with Cheese | 28 |

**Table 4:** The approximate fat content of single servings of some of the most popular fast food items derived from popular press. The fat is largely of the saturated type and the food may contain a relatively large amount of trans-fatty acids that may be dangerous to health. These fast food items are not much different in composition than many processed animal protein products that are found in all stores. Such data vary with time. Please note, not all "fast food" is unhealthy.

## "The Double Whopper Mentality"

It has been estimated that the average daily intake of fat has increased over the last decade up to an approximate average of 83 grams per day in adults. Fats are very efficient sources of unwanted calories. Who can really discuss the nutritional value of fast-food and "keep a straight face" (or belly) when one really examines examples of its calorie and fat content? (Table 4). America is engaged in the pleasurable pastime of "supersizing" its meals while the press reports the need for "supersizing" seats in public areas, in order to accommodate our expanded "rear ends". Please forgive the harshness, I need to overcome the complacency without being offensive. Later, I shall address the health dangers of "high saturated fat diets" for weight loss. These popular diets are not healthy in the long term, even though they may promote short-term weight loss in some people.

### Countering Complacency

In order to assist in countering the very powerful mental dynamics that an individual can use to deny a risk or reject a corrective lifestyle intervention, I have summarized with purpose the several ways of almost ensuring cardiovascular disease or premature death (Table 3). The keen eye will see that a cardiovascular risk is often equally a risk for other common killer diseases, e.g. cancer. These concepts lie at the basis of an effective combat against Syndrome X ( or X, Y and Z...) and other risk factors for disease. I do not wish to dwell on the sarcasm, but what is wrong is obvious, we just do not seem "to get the picture".

### Overcoming the Complacency About Syndrome X

Western nations face a health crisis in the form of Syndrome X. This crisis is amplified by a lack of clear definition and recognition of this powerful enemy against health. Syndrome X robs society of health and life in a pernicious, sinister and occult manner. It is relatively easy to vilify certain diseases, especially when they produce an overt effect or clear physical disability. For example, cancer conjures up ideas of "wasting away" and HIV disease is perceived as a nefarious illness with horrific outcome. In contrast, Syndrome X is not likely to provoke this kind of public reaction because of its widespread occurrence with manifestations that may breed complacency. After dinner conversations about one's weight or blood cholesterol are common and Syndrome X has a quiet, progressive nature that breeds on our complacency. Something that "kills you softly" may not provoke public revulsion or even major concern.

It should be recognized that an established pattern of Syndrome X carries similar threats, in terms of disability and risk of death, as does an initial diagnosis of many forms of cancer, HIV or other chronic killer diseases. Using HIV disease as an example, in many cases of HIV there is often a long incubation period following viral infection in which individuals enjoy relatively good health, before serious medical consequences of HIV emerge. By comparison, when Syndrome X is established, disability and death may occur in a similar time frame (about 10 years), interspersed with periods of variable ill health. HIV disease has been appropriately vilified, but lack of vilification of Syndrome X may tend to breed complacency and perhaps even medical inertia (failure of healthcare agencies and personnel to act).

A simple issue, that may cause Syndrome X to escape scrutiny by the public at large, is the fact that the variable occurrences of obvious manifestations of Syndrome X are so common (Figure 1) that they may be readily accepted as "normal" or even inevitable. In the US, we are not strangers to obesity, high blood cholesterol and hypertension with a pre-diabetic state, but we tend to think about these disorders alone and in isolation (or in a unitary manner). Clearly, it is better to view these disorders as a "gang of terrorists" that remove health and well-being. To remove the terror of Syndrome X means to remove the whole "gang of medical disorders", not just the most obvious, single, threatening "gang member". This is why just lowering cholesterol, just losing weight, just treating hypertension etc. will not do the trick. The components of Syndrome X are major risk factors that are making people "drop like flies" from cardiovascular disease.

## INSULIN RESISTANCE: THE MISCREANT

The root cause of Syndrome X appears to be resistance to the actions of insulin in the body. However, medical testing has not focused on the issue of the early diagnosis or clear recognition of insulin resistance. A diagnostic pronouncement of high blood cholesterol or high blood pressure is common place, but few individuals currently contemplate or discuss any new- found resistance to insulin. I believe that the sinister and pernicious nature of Syndrome X requires much more public education. With education will come appropriate vilification of this disorder and we may be able to overcome the persistent inertia that has existed to permit Syndrome X to persist among us in a relatively unchallenged manner.

## SYNDROME X: MUTINY OF THE TISSUES OF THE BODY

Dr. Gerald Reaven MD first labeled the cluster of risk factors in the metabolic syndrome as "Syndrome X" in 1988 (Table 2). At that time, he stressed that Syndrome X was caused by a large number of intertwined changes in body chemistry which were largely attributable to insulin resistance. Syndrome X is a medical conundrum where the command of the vital hormone insulin is not heeded. The insulin command is not taken by those cells of the body upon which this hormone exerts its maximum effects in terms of glucose uptake. When body tissues form a "mutiny" against the command of insulin, more insulin is poured out by the pancreas to overcome the disobedience. Mutiny comes in degrees of resilience and not all mutineers look alike. Thus, individuals have varying manifestations and degrees severity of Syndrome X.

This variability of insulin resistance and its consequences can be materially influenced by the genetic characteristics of an individual or their choice of lifestyle. Sorting out Syndrome X requires a multipronged approach which recognizes the complex interplay of all of the factors involved (Table 1 and 2). These factors work together to create the cardiovascular risks that attack our health and well-being. In this book, we shall examine each cardinal component of Syndrome X (high blood cholesterol, hypertension, obesity and insulin resistance or diabetes) and see how they "hang together". This dangerous gang of medical disorders can then be characterized and effectively tackled in a manner that will combat Syndrome X, or Syndrome X, Y and Z....

## Far Reaching Effects of Insulin

Insulin has many more jobs to do than just push glucose into cells. It is the complexities of the actions of insulin that are under active investigation, in order that we can understand how insulin resistance and excess evolves into Syndrome X or Syndrome X, Y and Z.... Actions of insulin, over and above its effects on sugar metabolism, broaden the significance of this disorder as a health risk beyond cardiovascular disease. For example, a complex interplay of insulin and other hormones leads to an association of Syndrome X with female hormonal disorders that result in the polycystic ovary syndrome, infertility, immune dysfunction and perhaps cancer or chronic inflammation in the body. Insulins' actions affect sugar, fat and protein metabolism in the body.

Whilst we recognize insulin as providing the primary signal to regulate glucose in the body, it also effects the storage and use of other basic nutrients in the body. Insulin has a tissue building effect by affecting mechanisms of the storage of carbohydrates, proteins and fats in cells. A deficiency of insulin can lead to breakdown of muscle protein. Insulin tends to exert most of its effects on tissues of the liver, muscles and fatty deposits, but it also acts on the growth and chemistry of many other tissues.

Insulin acts through receptors rather like a "lock and key" mechanism. Insulin is the "key" that fits into the "lock" (a receptor). When the insulin lock or receptor is activated, insulin goes about its complex duties. Thus, different locks (receptors) can be at fault and the function of insulin receptors may vary somewhat. The key may fit the lock but the lock may not turn. There are also variations in the "type" of insulin receptors. Examples of these variations of the receptors are called insulin-like growth factor I receptors (IGI-I).

The actions of insulin can be seen to be very complex, but it is important to know that multitude of actions of insulin exist through receptor stimulation. These actions alter the chemistry of the body that controls fats and proteins as well as glucose. Insulin is a trophic hormone (trophos=growth) causing tissue growth in some circumstances. This growth promoting effect of insulin may help to explain the relationship of hyperinsulinism, diabetes, obesity and Syndrome X with certain types of cancer. In addition to profound effects on enzymes (e.g. glycogen synthetase)in the body that make storage sugars (glycogen) from glucose, insulin affects transport of nutrients across cell membranes, enzymes involved in protein chemistry in the body and even the expressions of genes that conduct the chemistry of life.

## INSULIN RECEPTORS: THE LOCK AND THE KEY

Whilst most of our discussions have focussed on insulin resistance, this resistance is a function of both, the key (insulin) and the lock (the insulin receptor). Receptors for insulin go through their own changes in number and structure and their presence and functions are affected by many factors including genetics and lifestyle issues, as well as by insulin's presence itself ! In some circumstances, insulin receptors decrease in number when blood insulin levels increase in amount. This situation where insulin receptors decrease in number as a consequence of excess insulin may play a major role in the cause of insulin resistance itself. For example, this mechanism of the occurrence of a reduction or inactivity of receptors is the best explanation for the association of insulin resistance with obesity. One can now see just how complicated the evolution of the constellation of disorders within Syndrome X appears to be and how the significance of Syndrome X for health may extend way beyond cardiovascular risks! These facts support my concept of Syndrome X, Y and Z...

There are a whole host of diseases or conditions where the insulin receptors (the insulin lock) are altered in amount or function. Table 5 summarizes these circumstances. I accept that considerations of states of insulin sensitivity and insulin resistance are complex for the layperson, but it serves the purpose of showing how far–ranging the issues of insulin resistance are in terms of general health.

| States of insulin resistance | States of insulin sensitivity |
|---|---|
| Obesity | Anorexia nervosa |
| Maturity onset diabetes | Starvation |
| Growth hormone excess | Deficiency of growth hormone |
| Kidney disease resulting in renal failure | Loss of adrenal function, low cortisol |
| Liver disease, immune disorders, hereditary disorders | Drinking, drugs or natural products that enhance insulin sensitivity |

**Table 5**: Conditions where one can see changes in insulin receptor functions. These considerations broaden our understanding of the health implications of the changes in the actions of insulin.

## MECHANISMS OF INSULIN RESISTANCE

Suffice it to say, the exact causes of resistance to insulin remain only partially understood. These matters cannot be covered in detail in this book and they involve highly technical discussions. In summary, various mechanisms operate in controlling the functions of insulin in the body including: environmental factors, lifestyle issues, immune functions and genetics. Whilst we have to discuss the "unknown" to some degree, when considering the cause of insulin resistance, our knowledge of situations that make insulin resistance worse, or tend to precipitate or aggravate insulin resistance, is quite well defined. Insulin is a key player in what Dr. Claude Bernard discussed in the 19th century as his concept of the "reciprocal harmony" of life.

A number of medications can affect the secretion and or action of insulin and diseases or factors that tend to result in diabetes mellitus have been well defined. These issues are discussed in greater detail in Section 3 of this book. Table 6 lists many drugs that can alter glucose regulation in the body through effects on insulin. Table 6 is important to inspect in detail. The concept that "it may be your drugs" is of increasing importance as we worry more and more about iatrogenic (healthcare) induced disease. This type of disease, induced by healthcare interventions, kills more than 100,000 people per year in the US.

| Agents | Examples |
|---|---|
| Environmental chemicals | Fluoride, DDT, ethanol, cigarette smoking and pesticides |
| Hormones | Glucagon<br>Cortisol<br>Growth hormone<br>Sex hormones (contraceptive pill) |
| Drugs | Anticonvulsants e.g. phenytoin, diuretics e.g. thiazides, furosemide, Antiparasitic drugs e.g. pentamidine, Cancer chemotherapy e.g. L-asparaginase, mithramycin, antihypertensive drugs, beta blocker drugs, tranquilizers etc. |
| "Micronutrients" | Calcium, zinc, potassium, lithium, chromium, boron, cadmium and barium |

**Table 6:** Drugs or chemicals that may cause problems with or alter the actions of insulin and impact glucose control and Syndrome X. Note: some effects are desirable, others are not

## Syndrome "X, Y and Z..."

Whilst Syndrome X is a common and major risk for heart disease, stroke and peripheral vascular disease, I have stated repeatedly that it has other serious implications for health. This is why I have chosen to extend the concept of "Syndrome X" to "Syndrome X, Y and Z...".

Syndrome X is linked to insulin resistance, glucose intolerance and high blood glucose. This situation results in the generation of free radicals which cause oxidative stress to the body (see Section 8 for more complete description of oxidative damage to body tissues). With a rise in blood glucose, damaging free radicals contribute to the undesirable combination of glucose with cellular proteins to produce substances called "advanced glycation end-products" (AGES). The terms advanced glycation end-products (AGES) describe the end result of the combination of excessive glucose in the body with protein, in the presence of free radicals. The combining of glucose with protein refers to the terms "glycate" or "glycation".

The AGES generated by unwanted combinations of glucose and proteins (glycated products) can damage many body tissues. This damage often affects the tissues of the kidney, eyes and nervous system (organs commonly damaged in diabetic individuals). Free radical damage to tissues causes oxidative stress which has been associated with many types of chronic degenerative disease including arthritis, immune disorders, cardiovascular disease, inflammation, cancer and premature aging.

Table 7 summarizes the far reaching effects of insulin resistance that results in high blood glucose levels and, in turn, oxidative stress to body tissues.

| Medical Consequences of Glucose Intolerance | Comments |
| --- | --- |
| Oxidative stress to body tissues | When glucose is used as fuel, free radicals are generated in excess. |
|  | Oxidative damage occurs to all body systems and this causes premature aging. |
| Generation of "Advanced Glycation End-products" (AGES) | AGES damage many tissues in the body. e.g. kidneys, eyes, nerves. |
| Switching on of tricylyceride and LDL production | Abnormal blood fats (lipids) promote heart disease. High and more dense LDL and raised triglycerides. |

| | |
|---|---|
| Hypertension | By mechanisms not fully understood high blood pressure and its cardiovascular consequences occur (heart attack, stroke etc.). |
| Obesity | Insulin acts to increase fat deposition in the body. |
| Immune system damage | Oxidative stress and glucose itself interfere with key immune functions e.g. white cell function and antibody production. |
| Cancer increases | A clear link exists with womb (endometrial cancer) and obesity. Breast, colon, lung, prostate and gallbladder cancer may be linked with glucose intolerance or high insulin levels. |
| Polystic ovary syndrome (PCOS) | Insulin resistance is associated with PCOS, which causes masculinization, irregular menstruation and infertility. There is a suggestion that "feminization" occurs in males. |
| Premature aging | "AGES" and oxidative stress precipitate disease and tissue aging. |
| Switching eicosanoids | Switching in eicosanoid pathways, involving prostaglandins may promote inflammatory and cardiovascular disorders. |

| Change in eicosanoid actions | Essential fatty acids are directed into pathways that favor inflammation and blood clotting. This action occurs through pathways of prostaglandin metabolism promotion inflammatory disease, immune dysfunction, cancer, cardiovascular disease and cognitive decline (e.g. cerebrovascular disease and Alzheimers Disease). |

**Table 7:** The medical consequences of insulin resistance, glucose intolerance and diabetes are highlighted. The effects are far reaching and expand the risks of Syndrome X beyond cardiovascular disease to many other illnesses and premature death. These factors contribute to the concept of "Syndrome X, Y and Z..." proposed by the author.

## POLYCYSTIC OVARY SYNDROME (PCOS)

Whilst Syndrome X may be recognized inappropriately as a typical male trait, less focus has been placed on the special significance of Syndrome X and insulin resistance for young women. The typical individual with polycystic ovary syndrome (PCOS) is premenopausal and has obesity, excess body hair, irregular menstruation, acne and infertility. This syndrome is sometimes called the Stein-Leventhal syndrome, named after the two physicians who discovered this disorder, without knowing its cause. The pivotal cause of this problem is insulin resistance and polycystic ovary syndrome has been referred to as "Syndrome X of the ovaries". In addition, the temporary presence of glucose intolerance in pregnancy, known as "Gestational Diabetes", is an example of Syndrome X of pregnancy.

To recognize the association of PCOS as part of Syndrome X further reinforces the far reaching health consequences of the metabolic changes that occur with insulin resistance. As the name suggest the PCOS results in multiple cysts in the ovary. The relationship between insulin secretion and female hormonal status and ovarian function is complex. In simple terms, the excess circulating insulin that occurs as a consequence of insulin resistance (Syndrome X) stimulates special cells in the ovary (theca cells) to produce excesses of male-type hormones (testosterone); and it upsets the function of the pituitary gland that secretes hormones that regulate menstrual cycles and gonadal functions (sexual organ functions). Excess male hormones cause excessive body hair of a male pattern of distribution and alters the menstrual cycle of young women with PCOS.

## TECHNICAL NOTES (FOR HEALTHCARE GIVERS)

Not everyone in conventional medical practice has "bought in" to the significance of the links among the combination features of Syndrome X. For many years, physicians have debated the characteristic features of a metabolic syndrome where obesity, hypertension and hyperlipidemia go hand in hand with glucose intolerance. This cluster of conditions has been termed Syndrome X or the "metabolic syndrome" where resistance to the actions of insulin appear to be the primary metabolic defect, according to Dr. G. Reaven MD and others.

The terms "Syndrome X" have been criticized and some physicians have preferred to talk exclusively in terms of the "metabolic syndrome". There is no doubt that terms have been confusing as earlier references to Syndrome X in medical literature were used to describe microangiopathy of the myocardium (microvascular disease, especially found in diabetes) and even confused with Prinzmetal's-Angina (variant angina described in 1908, by Myron Prinzmental MD), or types of syncope or headache. Dr. Gerald Reaven MD did not have these disorders in mind when he described his killer cardiovascular risk cluster of Syndrome X, which he believes to be fundamentally related to insulin resistance.

Syndrome X is a disease with a relatively indistinct definition because modern research is still uncovering the potential far reaching significance of states of insulin resistance. This is why I felt justified in expanding terminology to "Syndrome X, Y and Z…". I believe that the various components of Syndrome X may have independent expression and their separate identity (polygenic nature) is clouded by common adverse lifestyle factors, most notably poor nutrition. However, modern research shows that type 2 diabetes mellitus is often preceded by a period of time in which insulin resistance is measurable, especially in terms of the measurable resistance of muscle cells to the actions of insulin.

It has been argued that the combination of obesity and insulin resistance (a sine quo non of common forms of Syndrome X) is not in itself an adequate explanation for the pathogenesis of Type 2 diabetes. There appears to be a need for malfunction of beta cells that secrete insulin. This argument does not defeat the notion that insulin resistance may be the most important pre-monitory event in the escalating incidence of type 2 diabetes mellitus. Furthermore, the picture seems to be clearer in maturity onset diabetes in the young (MODY), where mutation of the glucokinase gene is well described. There are a host of genes of varying significance that affect insulin action or secretion in the presence or absence of obesity or adverse lifestyle. These genes are drug targets and their function is regulated by intrinsic metabolic changes e.g. eicosanoid status. Regulation of PPAR genes by eicosapentanoic acid (EPA) is a very interesting new observation (see Section 8).

First degree relatives of patients with type 2 diabetes and longitudinal studies of prediabetic individuals show that hyperinsulinemia and insulin resis-tance is often concomitant. Furthermore, clear relationships have been defined between the presence of hyperinsulinemia and the development of hyperten-sion, certain forms of dyslipidemias and premature cardiovascular disease. Obesity figures strongly in the equations of cardiovascular risk, especially in the "pot bellied" person (centripetal obesity). These findings are well docu-mented in many scientific papers which form an essential background to the understanding of the notions that I express. Whilst the precise metabolic defects that cause insulin resistance require further elucidation, lifestyle change (diet and exercise) are now appreciated as pivotal in preventing the combination of disorders within Syndrome X.

## CHAPTER SUMMARY

Syndrome X is characterized by underlying resistance to the actions of the hormone insulin. Insulin resistance is a state where a given amount of insulin in the body produces less than a desirable effect on body tissues. This circumstance leads to a chain of altered events in body chemistry that favors the occurrence of poor sugar balance, obesity, high blood cholesterol and hypertension. These are the cardinal components of Syndrome X which cause cardiovascu-lar disease – the number one killer in Western society (Figure 1).

The actions of insulin are much broader than the regulation of glucose handling by the body. Syndrome X can impact repro-ductive function and other health issues. These observations under-lie my expanded concept of "Syndrome X" to "Syndrome X, Y and Z..." The key to the combat of Syndrome X is an understanding of the interplay of each component of the Syndrome, against the pivotal issue of insulin resistance, and the use of inter- ventions that will address all of the aspects of the combination of disorders within Syndrome X. To date, no allopathic intervention has come close to addressing the global problem of Syndrome X or Syndrome X, Y and Z...

# SECTION 2

# COMBAT CHOLESTEROL: WHEN THE TREATMENT MAY BE WORSE THAN THE DISEASE

## HUMOR THAT IS NOT FUNNY

The gamblers among us may have a sure bet, if they back the likelihood of the giving a prescription for a cholesterol-lowering-medication following a periodic health examination in a mature American. It has been stated sarcastically, in medical circles, that such a prescription may be written before the medical consultation, if the patients' blood tests are available prior to the examination by the treating physician. No blame can be apportioned in this occasional "folie a deux" which merely represents the fulfillment of a patient's learned expectations by a physician who wishes to comply with "standards of care", even if such standards are nebulous. That said, "never a truer word has been said in jest".

## THE FOLLY OF JUST LOWERING CHOLESTEROL, JUST LOSING WEIGHT ETC

Focusing only on one component of Syndrome X or one cardiovascular risk factor is short sighted. All the risks with Syndrome X and the "bouquet of barbed wire" need to be addressed together if we are to combat Syndrome X and reverse its contributions to premature death. Some well conducted clinical trials have failed to show a clear connection between dietary, saturated fat and cholesterol intake and the development of coronary artery disease or "hardening of the arteries" (atheroma). On the other hand, there are many more studies that have indicated that a clear connection exists. This situation is at least very confusing, but it is readily explained. "Just" lowering cholesterol is not enough to reduce risks of heart disease. All risk factors need to be tackled, together!

## Applying Lifestyle Interventions: Addressing All Issues

Some studies that examine the reversal of the risks of heart disease have included several beneficial lifestyle interventions, in addition to dietary changes. For example lowering cholesterol and lowering saturated fat intake in the diet with added fiber and restricted salt are known to be healthy interventions. If multiple beneficial interventions are studied together in one clinical trial, then it is difficult to factor out the significance of one particular intervention, such as a low-cholesterol or low-fat diet alone. The situation is complex when one considers that "low-fat" diets may often be "high-carbohydrate" diets in disguise. I reiterate that there has been an obsession in modern research of defining one risk factor in isolation of the others. This approach is perhaps necessary to satisfy a defined burden of scientific proof, but it causes confusion among the public and firmly molds the practice of some physicians.

It is clear from modern research that impacting all aspects of Syndrome X is the way to go. Since insulin resistance is the main underlying cause of Syndrome X and its cardiovascular consequences, the disturbed body chemistry triggered by this resistance and compensatory excess of insulin (hyperinsulinism) must be addressed. High blood levels insulin which occur as a result of insulin resistance switch on the production of damaging fats (types of cholesterol) in the body. I shall explore some good reasons to question the effectiveness of a narrow focus on cholesterol reduction by drugs, as an effective strategy for reducing the risk of coronary artery disease and other consequences of arteriosclerosis (atheroma, clogging of arterial blood vessels).

## Advantages of Combating Multiple Risk Factors

The failure of focused medicals interventions to reduce cardiovascular (CVS) disease is apparent in the Multiple Risk Factor

Intervention Trial (MRFT) that was undertaken in the mid-1970's. This clinical trial examined the role of reducing dietary cholesterol and saturated fats as a means of preventing heart disease. This study found that these interventions were less successful than may have been initially anticipated. The MRFT involved the study of approximately 12,000 men who were considered at risk from cardiovascular disease. This group of men were divided into two groups, where one group was advised to take a diet designed to reduce blood cholesterol levels and the other group were given no advice about specific dietary interventions.

In both groups normal supportive medical care occurred, such as the prescription of medication to reduce blood pressure. This prospective (forward, ongoing) study showed that the group who were advised to take a low cholesterol diet were able to achieve overall lower serum cholesterol values and lower blood pressure recordings than the group who did not receive a specific dietary intervention. However, no improvement in death rate from cardiovascular disease was noted as a consequence of the dietary intervention alone to lower cholesterol. The presence of the complex "bouquet of barbed wire" of cardiovascular risks and the folly of examining a focused intervention explains the apparent negative outcome of the MRFT.

## EXTREMES OF OPINION ENTER THE PICTURE

Some researchers have gone further in their criticism of "channeled", medical interventions to lower cholesterol. These individuals have questioned the use of drugs to lower serum cholesterol and some "nutritionally-orientated" physicians have described the practice of lowering blood cholesterol with drug therapy as perhaps worthless and quite dangerous! This polar opinion seems to be unjustified and the answer lies somewhere between the extremes of opinion. There are many cardiovascular risk factors (see Syndrome X and the X factors (Figure 1, Tables 1 and 2, Section 1) that are inextricably linked in the causation of atheroma (clogging arteries) or atherosclerosis (hardening of the arteries). In addition, other risks for coronary artery disease form the "bouquet of barbed wire" (Section 1). Attempting to focus on one risk factor alone at the expense of considering the synergistic, adverse health effects of all risk factors, is an all too common mistake in current medical practice. I belabor this issue because it is holding us back in our fight against Syndrome X and cardiovascular disease.

I must emphasize that I do not believe that the lowering of blood cholesterol is an unnecessary pastime. However, this intervention must be undertaken with a "multi-pronged" approach to cardiovascular and other disease prevention by addressing all risk factors in a simultaneous manner. Opinions that abnormalities of blood cholesterol are not part of the cause of cardiovascular problems should be rejected; with the added caveat that high blood cholesterol is only one of several major components of cardiovascular risk factors (Tables 1 and 2, Section 1).

## Who Owns the Cardiovascular Risk Factors?

To perceive that an individual is not the owner of his or her own cardiovascular risk (CVS) factors is a common, self-styled deception. Whilst there are risk factors, such as "genetic gifts" or "gender" that are unchangeable, most cardiovascular risk factors can be changed for the better. Even if an individual has established heart disease or atherosclerosis, there are many ways to prevent advancing disease that are within the control of the individual. It is never too late in life to use preventive strategies against Syndrome X and ensuing cardiovascular disease.

Advancing age is not considered to be an independent risk factor for cardiovascular disease. Few people would argue with the statistical observation that the older one becomes, the greater the risk of coronary artery disease, but several scientific studies have suggested that lowering cholesterol in the "mature adult" can lower the risk of coronary heart disease. Chronological age does not always coincide with biological age. We are all aware of the 40-year-old man in the 70-year-old body and vice versa. There are several readily identifiable risk factors that can be ameliorated and many bear a direct or indirect relationship to the problem of high blood cholesterol (Table 10). Equally, there are several simple goals that underlie attempts to make such changes (Table 10).

| Cardiovascular risk factors amenable to change: | Aims of a simple CVS risk factor reduction program: |
| --- | --- |
| Obesity | Achieve and or maintain ideal body weight |
| High blood cholesterol | Decrease saturated fat and simple sugar intake |
| High blood pressure | Reduce sodium intake |
| Smoking | Stop smoking |
| Physical inertia | Exercise |
| Low levels of high density lipoprotein | Nutritional changes, exercise |
| Prevention of diabetes mellitus * | Weight control, exercise and nutrition |

**Table 10:** Cardiovascular risk factors that are readily changed and simple approaches to reducing risks(*). In 2001, the Diabetes Prevention Program in the US confirmed that exercise and weight reduction may prevent maturity onset diabetes mellitus. Maturity onset diabetes is often preceded by insulin resistance, a pivotal component of Syndrome X. Furthermore, in the summer of 2001, the Secretary of Human Health Services of the US announced a large investment of funds to educate the public on diabetes prevention (essentially an attack on Syndrome X).

## OVERLOOKING DIET AS THE KEY TO CARDIOVASCULAR HEALTH

Several options exist for the reduction of blood cholesterol, including diet, exercise, the addition of fractions of soluble fiber (beta glucans) in the diet, alteration of the type of protein consumed in the diet (e.g. vegetable versus meat protein), increasing omega 3 fatty acid intake and drug therapy. There has been an exponential increase in the use of cholesterol lowering drugs in clinical practice, but such drugs are expensive, associated with unpleasant side effects, and, on occasion, they can be frankly dangerous (Table 11). The main type of synthetic pharmaceuticals that are used for their cholesterol-lowering effects and their adverse effects are shown in Table11. These drugs are are often overused in conventional medical practice at the expense of considering or exhausting lifestyle and dietary adjustments as first line options.

| Class/Drug | Action | Side Effects |
|---|---|---|
| Bile acid sequestrants Cholestyramine Colestipol | Remove bile acids from enterohepatic circulation lowers LDL by 15-30% | Gastrointestinal distress, constipation, Interference with drug and nutrient absorption |
| Nicotinic acid | Inhibits secretion of lipoproteins by liver, modest changes in LDL, VLDL, and HDL | Only tolerated by 50% of patients because of gastrointestinal distress, flushing, itching, skin rash, liver toxicity and gout |
| HMG CoA reductase inhibitors Lovastatin Provastatin Simvastatin "The Statins" | Inhibit cholesterol synthesis in liver, lower LDL by 25%-35%, raise HDL by 10% (sometimes) | Expensive, abnormal liver function, sometimes serious. Need monitoring of liver function. Myopathy and weakness, occasional deaths. |
| Fibric acids Clofibrate Gemfibrizol | Increase activity of lipoprotein lipase and lower triglycerides Modest effect only on LDL and HDL | Gastrointestinal distress, cause of gallstones and myopathy (severe sometimes, occasionally fatal) |

| Probucol | Lowers LDL and protects LDL against oxidation, but lowers HDL | Gastrointestinal distress. Lowering HDL is dangerous. Prevention of heart disease not well documented |
|---|---|---|

**Table 11: Cholesterol-Lowering Drugs. All are expensive, sometimes** costing in excess of $120 for a month's treatment, and they have troublesome side effects. Adverse effects of these drugs may be sometimes dose dependent so that a natural option that could limit dosage requirements would be a real advantage (see soy, omega 3 fatty acids, soluble fiber and beta glucan extracts of soluble fiber, Section 7). The abbreviation HMG CoA stands for hydroxymethylglutaryl coenzyme A, a liver enzyme involved in cholesterol synthesis that is inhibited by "statin-type" drugs and by-products of soluble fiber.

THE FIRST LINE OPTION IS NOT A DRUG

The public have been somewhat "brain-washed" with the idea that the road to lowering blood cholesterol is the ideal, and perhaps only, pathway to cardiovascular health. This road is not "a yellow-brick road". No doubt, concerns about high blood cholesterol create niggling doubts in many peoples' minds. Furthermore, fewer and fewer middle-aged individuals get the reassurance of a low blood cholesterol result during periodic health examination. Despite the anxiety about high blood cholesterol, medical approaches are often limited to dietary advice about reducing fat and cholesterol intake, sometimes combined with a "premature" prescription or recommendation for a lipid-lowering drug.

There is an enthusiastic willingness of a physician to adopt a pharmacological (drug) approach to the therapy of high blood cholesterol and an equal willingness for the person with a high blood cholesterol to take this "apparent" easy way out, by filling their drug prescription (purchase order). Healthcare revenues are skewed towards drug prescriptions, not lifestyle advice. I stress that lowering cholesterol and simultaneous enhancement of general health by good lifestyle and nutrition is the ideal, "first–line" approach for many people.

Media advertising of cholesterol-lowering drugs tends to focus on the failure of diet and exercise to work and encourage the drug option. This media message does not encourage the correct first line option. The "drug–free" approach can often be effective, but it requires commitment. Gentle, natural approaches are preferable "first line-options" for many health-conscious individual who want to control blood cholesterol and impact the other cardinal components of Syndrome X. Fortunately, these issues are becoming more recognized as the general public is demanding increasingly that general health be promoted through "natural" and/or nutritional means.

## PREMATURE PRESCRIPTION PRACTICE?

Several multinational pharmaceutical companies have developed cholesterol-lowering drugs as a consequence of the widespread nature of the problem of hypercholesterolemia (high blood cholesterol) and the lucrative prospects in this area of healthcare. Studies have emerged which show that physicians may be apt to prescribe synthetic cholesterol-lowering drugs without exhausting the possibility of more natural means of lowering blood cholesterol. It may be that many patients are being placed at unnecessary risk from these drugs. Several studies have demonstrated that special "diets" combined with lifestyle changes are highly effective not only in reducing blood cholesterol but also in causing a variable regression in atherosclerotic disease. For example, Dr. Dean Ornish (1990) has proposed an effective, holistic program involving diet and lifestyle change to improve cardiovascular health. Such programs can now be modified to be even more effective in light of our knowledge about ideal nutritional and/or nutraceutical approaches to Syndrome X. In contrast, several findings question the cost-effectiveness of drugs for cholesterol lowering.

## DANGERS AND DISADVANTAGES OF CHOLESTEROL LOWERING DRUGS

I have proposed that targeted drug therapy to "just" lower blood cholesterol in isolation may be short-sighted or even "foolish" medicine. Equally, cholesterol reduction achieved solely by the dietary exclusion of saturated fat, sugar or cholesterol and synthetic lipid lowering drugs, in the absence of a nutritional program to improve general health, is not always safe and it is not cost-effective. These approaches do not take into account the many components of Syndrome X that create a serious risk for cardiovascular diseases. The ability of cholesterol lowering drugs to reduce cholesterol, the "easy way", has made effort-requiring, dietary approaches unattractive and it has overshadowed the importance of drug side-effect profiles. Perhaps one could argue that the perceived "easy way out" with a cholesterol lowering drug may function to give a sense of security which then promotes adverse lifestyle that, in turn, causes an elevation of blood cholesterol?

I have stated repeatedly that side effects of lipid lowering drugs are sometimes serious and such drugs are expensive. The most popular type of cholesterol lowering drugs are the "statin type". "Statin" drugs interfere with liver enzymes (HMG CoA reductase) that play a key role in cholesterol production in the body. In Section 7 of this book, some readers may be surprised to learn that beta glucan fractions of oat soluble fiber may have a mechanism of action similar to a statin drug, without the side effects. Some of the disadvantages of "statin-type" drugs are highlighted in Table 12. There are clear and overriding reasons to seek safer, natural options to lower cholesterol, normalize blood lipids and promote general wellness, especially by using natural approaches to reduce the occurrence of the components of Syndrome X. In summary, cholesterol lowering drugs are expensive, often associated with side effects, not suitable for growing children or teenagers and they are sometimes frankly dangerous (Table 12).

- Expense
- Compliance problems
- Common liver problems requiring cessation of therapy
- Occasional severe muscle disorders
- Cannot be used in children.

- Deplete Co-enzyme Q10 which is energizing and required for cardiovascular and central nervous system health.
- Long term side effects unknown
- General, variable side effects e.g. headache, gastrointestinal side effects etc.
- Drug interactions
- Occasional deaths

**Table 12**: Problems with "statin type" drugs. Note: Other popular cholesterol-lowering drugs may have serious side effects.

In many cases the long-term effects of drug therapy to reduce cholesterol, especially statin-type drugs, is unknown. A specific statin drug was removed from the market in the summer of 2001 because it caused deaths. Although recent studies claim a reduction in heart attacks with the use of certain cholesterol lowering drugs, there is no "substantial" evidence that the overall death rate from heart attacks can be "substantially" reduced by this limited pharmacological (drug) approach.

## STATIN DRUGS ARE FOR HIGH RISKS ONLY

Whilst the interest in using "statin" drugs becomes frenetic, important studies that show the limited cost–effectiveness of these drugs have passed unnoticed. When one examines contemporary scientific studies that examine the cost effectiveness of cholesterol-lowering therapies along with specific characteristics of patients with high blood cholesterol, the limitations of "statins" become obvious.

Dr. L. Prosser MD and colleagues show that statin drug therapy is not cost universally effective, except in people with high risks such as the presence of established heart disease (Prosser LA, Stinnett, AA, Goldman PA and colleagues Ann. Int. Med, 132, 769-79, 2000). This important study concluded that the prevention of cardiovascular with a statin type drug was not cost effective for healthy young men or women who did not have high risk factors for cardiac disease. Other studies support these conclusions.

A nutritional program that can effectively reduce cholesterol and impact Syndrome X has many other associated health benefits. Specific nutritional agents that lower cholesterol and combat aspects of Syndrome X, in addition to high blood cholesterol, (e.g. special beta glucan components of soluble fiber, fish oil, soy and other phytonutrients) are generally safe and often cheaper than drug therapy. With nutritional programs, overall promotion of general wellness may occur. By this approach, one can address the dangers of Syndrome X or Syndrome X, Y and Z...

## REINFORCING THE CONCEPT OF
## COMBAT SYNDROME X (X, Y AND Z...)

At the same time that the public awareness was increasing in the cholesterol - heart disease link in the 1980's, some farsighted individuals attempted to promote what they termed "life extension" programs. The idea of life extension is neither novel nor new, since it has been a relatively unfulfilled ambition of humankind from early civilizations to the present. However, the real importance of life extension philosophies is that they broaden ideas to the concept of general wellness promotion rather than a fixation on only one part of a "health puzzle". Whilst Syndrome X has a clear role in the development of cardiovascular disease, it has even greater implications for health including altered menstruation, infertility and the propagation of cancer or inflammatory disease (perhaps through its effects on eicosanoid production). This is the broader concept of Syndrome X, Y and Z..."

I believe that the focus on cholesterol and cardiovascular risk has led to an unhealthy preoccupation of reducing only one risk factor for premature cardiovascular mortality (death) at the expense of the individual's consideration of more general health promotion. Again, the value of the concept of attacking the killer constellation of risks within Syndrome X becomes apparent. The terrorism tactics of Syndrome X result in silent progression to death and like any form of terrorism in our world today, we cannot choose one target and hope to eradicate the problem. The concept of impacting all factors that comprise Syndrome X is as justified as the concept of Syndrome X itself; and it reinforces the importance of the broadened concepts of combating Syndrome X, Y and Z....

## Examining the Cholesterol Theory

At the outset, it must be recognized that lowering blood cholesterol is advantageous for most people, but lowering cholesterol "alone" without consideration of other lifestyle or health concerns is not a worthy objective. In this context, the "cholesterol theory" of disease causation should be examined in some detail. Medical science has focused on high blood cholesterol as a principal contributing factor to a variety of diseases. The focus has rested most notably on a variety of cardiovascular diseases including: heart attack, stroke, peripheral vascular disease, arteriosclerosis and vascular causes of dementia. Other common and serious diseases may be associated with hypercholesterolemia (high blood cholesterol) including prostatic disease, renal diseases, pancreatic disease and certain cancers. This association operates through Syndrome X, Y and Z. . .

## Elevated Blood Homocysteine

The "homocysteine theory" of heart disease represents a different and important view of the cause of cardiovascular disease. Homocysteine is an amino acid that is produced through the breakdown of other proteins in the body. The essential amino acid, methionine, found in a variety of animal proteins, is indirectly the source of homocysteine. Homocysteine normally is present in very low concentrations because it is converted to another breakdown product, cystathionine, but please do not get bogged down in these terms. High levels of homocysteine in the body have been linked to arteriosclerosis and atheroma. In addition, high levels of homocysteine are also linked with increased blood-clotting activity in the body (an important member of the X-factors, Table 2, Section 2)..

In an uncommon congenital (hereditary) condition called homocysteinuria, the body lacks an enzyme to break down and metabolize certain proteins and hence, the blood contains abnormally high levels of homocysteine. These enzyme deficiencies have been noted in certain types of mental retardation, and homocysteinuria has been linked with premature cardiac death of children with this uncommon hereditary disease. One piece of the homocysteine puzzle emerged when severe coronary artery disease was found to be present in these children. These were, by the way, "incidental findings" arising from research into possible enzyme deficiencies as a causal factor in mental retardation. This information was first noted in research conducted in Northern Ireland in the 1960s, but its significance has only recently become clear (McCully KS, McCully M, The Heart Revolution, Harper Collins Publishers, NY, NY, 2000).

The link between elevated homocysteine levels among a small group of young children and the progression of heart disease in the general population was discovered in a process that reads like a complex medical "whodunit." Starting in the late 1960s and into the 1970s, research pathologist Kilmer McCully, M.D. gathered together what was known about homocysteine and homocysteinuria, conducted independent research, and eventually the important link between elevated homocysteine levels and the presence of atherosclerosis.

A key piece of the puzzle involves the role of B vitamins (folic acid vitamin B6 and B12) in metabolizing homocysteine and efficiently preventing high levels of homocysteine from accumulating in the body. For example, an animal study conducted in 1949 had demonstrated that a diet adequate in all ways, except for a deficiency in vitamin B6, led to atherosclerosis and a corresponding high level of homocysteine. Additional animal research and added to the body of evidence that established that high levels of homocysteine are implicated in the development of heart disease. Predictably, Dr. McCully's early findings were rejected by medical opinion, largely because it was promoted inappropriately as a challenge, rather than a complement, to the "cholesterol theory" of heart disease. When one puts one's head above the pulpit of medical opinion, it will be smacked with a "medical bible". Over the next couple of decades, other researchers eventually linked deficiencies of folic acid, B12, and B6 with high blood homocysteine levels and the progression of atheroma.

It is important to understand that the homocysteine theory, which could be called "the high blood levels of homocysteine" theory, is not in direct opposition to the cholesterol theory of heart disease, but rather helps to complete a picture of the link between diet and heart disease. It helps to explain why, in part, heart attacks may occur even when cholesterol levels are low and blood pressure is normal. This is illustrated in a study in which a group of Swedish researchers examined men under the age of fifty-five years who, prior to a first heart attack, had no warning signs that heart disease was present (i.e., they did not have high cholesterol levels or hypertension). The common link between these men was elevated homocysteine levels and correspondingly reduced blood levels of folic acid, along with levels of B12 in the lower end of the normal range.

Elevated blood homocysteine levels have been linked with increased risk of stroke and of peripheral arterial disease, a condition in which arteriosclerosis affects the arteries in the brain and extremities. It is known that more folic acid, vitamin B12 and vitamin B6 in the diet help to lower elevated blood levels of homocysteine. Improving the diet to increase dietary intake of these vitamins will tend to improve cardiovascular health; and when these nutrients are combined are with soluble fiber, beta glucans or say protien, a cocktail that promotes a healthy blood cholesterol and homocysteine level is produced (see Section 7, Syndrome X Nutritional Factors™).

## CLOGGING ARTERIES: HOW DOES ATHEROMA FORM IN BLOOD VESSELS?

The hallmark of hardening or "clogging" of blood vessels (atheroma) is the development of cholesterol containing plaque (fatty heaps) in the linings and walls of arteries in the body. It appears that injury to the lining of the blood vessel (artery) and excesses of circulating LDL (low density lipoprotein cholesterol, "bad" cholesterol) play a major role in the causation of the atheromatous plaques. It is "oxidized" LDL that is particularly prone to be deposited in arteries causing atheroma (plaque deposition). Furthermore, insulin resistance in Syndrome X tends to result in the production of a particularly damaging "dense-types" of LDL by the body. Injury to the lining of blood vessels may occur as a consequence of several factors, including diabetes mellitus, high blood pressure, smoking and immune mechanisms. One can see how the many components of Syndrome X combine together to compound cardiac risk. Therefore, any approach to these problems must be versatile, it cannot be focused on one issue (intentional echolalia).

## "CLOGGED ARTERIES"

Lipids (fats and cholesterol) are transported through the body in several formats. It is the deposition of these lipids from the LDL and VLDL (bad cholesterol) packages in the blood that leads to arterial blockage. Arteries throughout the body have many branches with decreasing diameters. For example, the internal diameter of a major human coronary artery ( artery supplying the heart muscle) is about 2-3 millimeters (1/12 of an inch) and it is easily clogged by heaps of fatty material (plaque), made up of bad types of cholesterol.

The mechanisms whereby lipids are deposited in arteries to cause atheroma have been increasingly understood in the past decade. It appears that lesions in the lining of arteries (intima) form foci for the deposition of cholesterol from LDL. Repair proteins, platelet aggregation, calcium deposition and additional fats aggregate over a long period of time to cause a buildup leading to arterial blockage. It is known that the development of clogged arteries is favored by the presence of high blood pressure and insulin resistance with glucose intolerance (diabetes mellitus). As we understand the interplay of these factors, the concept of syndrome X and the complex "battle plan" for its potential combat emerges with greater clarity.

"Damming up" of arteries can occur over a long period of time without symptoms. The first manifestation of its presence can be an acute heart attack with sudden death, with or without prior symptoms. The blockage of the blood vessels supplying the heart (coronary arteries) results in a starvation of oxygen and nutrients to the heart. This can cause the condition of angina pectoris where the heart "screams out in pain", due to a lack of blood supply. Angina pectoris is chest pain derived from lack of blood supply to the heart. Anginal chest pain occurs most often if exercise or physiological stresses place a demand for increased blood supply to the heart. This increased blood flow to the heart cannot occur because of the reduction of diameter and relaxability of the arteries.

The stiffening and clogging of arteries is caused by atheroma (plaque depositions with associated "hardening" of arteries). Whilst the events described are common in heart disease, a significant proportion of heart attacks may occur without classic symptoms, but with serious outcome. Recent studies have examined the outcome of "silent heart attacks" with a conclusion that they have the same serious consequences as heart attacks that occur with typical symptoms. A further risk in Syndrome X is the occurrence of a tendency for people to have easy blood clotting. When small clots form on atheromatous plaques in arteries they form an unstable deposit called "unstable plaque". Accelerated production of cholesterol by the liver in the presence of insulin resistance (Syndrome X) results in rapid accumulation of unstable plaque in arteries that causes clogging or can "break off" and block vessels (embolism). These circumstances in Syndrome X contribute to and compound cardiovascular events like heart attack and stroke.

## TYPES AND AMOUNTS OF BLOOD LIPIDS

The importance of hypercholesterolemia in the causation of coronary artery disease, peripheral vascular disease (poor circulation to the extremities of the body), and cerebrovascular disease (stroke) is well documented. Abnormalities in blood lipids (fats), including high blood cholesterol levels, are determined by complex factors, but poor diet frequently makes a significant contribution to this problem. This has led to recommendations by leading authorities (American Heart Association and the National Cholesterol Education Program) that dietary fat be reduced to 30 percent of the total daily intake of calories and fat of animal origin (saturated fat) should be limited. However, this advice from these leading bodies needs to be reexamined in the light of the importance of Syndrome X and Dr. Reaven's (and other's) advice on more liberal intake of "healthy" types of fat.

These days, we know that not all fat is bad and some is good for the heart. Good fat includes the unsaturated types of fat, most specifically omega-3 fatty acids that are found in certain plants (flax, canola or soy) and in fish oil. Furthermore, nutritionists have started to propose more liberal "good" fat intake in the diet as part of a diet for Syndrome X (see Sections 5 and 10). Fat does not tend to promote insulin secretion by the pancreas and this may help variably in the situation of insulin resistance. In addition, omega 3 fatty acids seem to combat insulin resistance. The main types of lipids (fats) found in the blood are summarized in Table 13.

| Lipoprotein | Major Lipid | Origin / F unction |
|---|---|---|
| Chylomicrons | Triglycerides | Transport of dietary fat from intestine |
| Bad Cholesterol Very low-density lipoprotein (VLDL) | Triglycerides | Transport from liver of endogenous fat |
| Bad Cholesterol Low-density lipoprotein (LDL) | Cholesterol | Liver, transport of cholesterol to peripheral tissue |
| Good Cholesterol High-density lipoprotein (HDL) | Cholesterol | Liver, Gut. Reverse cholesterol transport |

**Table 13**: Major Serum Lipoproteins (lipids, blood fats). LDL and VLDL are commonly referred as "bad" types of cholesterol, whereas HDL is referred to as a "good" type of cholesterol.

## DIFFERENT BLOOD FATS TO CONSIDER

The latter half of the 20th century has seen an ever-increasing number of scientific articles that clearly document the relationship between high blood cholesterol and heart disease; and newer research has shown that cholesterol is not the only type of blood fat (lipid) to consider. Prevention of coronary artery disease is possible with interventions that lower specific types of blood lipids (fats), not necessary all types of blood fats. Overall, it is believed that a high total blood cholesterol, a high low-density lipoprotein (LDL), a high very low-density lipoprotein level (VLDL), a high triglyceride level (TG), and a low high-density cholesterol level (HDL) are all deleterious to health. In Syndrome X, high LDL and triglycerides are encountered frequently. Indeed, high blood triglycerides are one of the "hallmarks" of Syndrome X. In simple terms, low-density cholesterol (LDL) is the bad type of cholesterol and high-density cholesterol (HDL) is the good type of cholesterol.

## PATTERNS OF HIGH BLOOD CHOLESTEROL

Varying abnormalities in total cholesterol, LDL, VLDL and HDL can be classified into certain types of high blood lipid patterns, or hyperlipoproteinemia. This classification is important because it has implications concerning the selection of therapy. However, the implications of this classification are more relevant when considering drug therapy to lower blood cholesterol because tailored nutritional interventions (e.g. soluble fiber, beta glucan fractions of soluble fiber, soy protein and fish oil) are often portable to most types of hyperlipoproteinemia (high blood cholesterol and fats). At the risk of over-simplification of the issues, the reader can conveniently remember that high density lipoprotein (HDL) is the only "good type of cholesterol"; essentially, the rest are bad!

## BAD CHOLESTEROL

Cholesterol is only one of several types lipids (fats) with variable functions that are found in the blood and tissues. Some understanding of the components of blood lipids is required in order to interpret abnormalities. Low density lipoproteins (LDL) are believed to be the major problem in determining atheroma and, in particular, coronary artery disease. Therefore, LDL is the "bad type" of cholesterol. In general, the higher the LDL the greater the risk of occurrence of coronary artery disease, but dense and oxidized forms of LDL are particularly damaging. In Syndrome X, the body also "churns" out damaging amounts of triglycerides, another form of "bad fat" in the blood and the type of LDL formed is of a "dense and damaging type".

## BAD CHOLESTEROL MADE WORSE

Low density lipoproteins carry cholesterol in the bloodstream. When LDL is oxidized, it is more likely to be deposited in the lining of arterial vessels leading to atheroma. Oxidized LDL (and peroxidated polyunsaturated fats) enhance atheroma formation (clogging of arteries). Natural ways to combat the oxidation of bad cholesterol (LDL) are very valuable in preventing heart disease. This can be achieved by taking dietary components that are rich in antioxidant components e.g. fruits, vegetables and certain minerals or vitamins etc. For this reason, certain forms of soluble fiber (guar gum, soy fiber and beta glucans) that are versatile in combating Syndrome X are enriched with antioxidants in useful dietary supplements (www.combatsyndromex.com), (see Sections 7 and 8). Furthermore, certain types of antioxidants, such as alpha lipoic acid and carnosine, are particularly valuable in preventing the formation of advanced glycation end products (AGES) and they help to prevent complications of diabetes (see Section 8).

Oxidized forms of cholesterol are atherogenic, that is they tend to cause cholesterol deposits that clog blood vessels. One must also consider the "trans-types" of fatty acids which seem to be very damaging. These types of fatty acids (components of fat) enter our diet when the healthy types of unsaturated fats are chemically treated (hydrogenated) in food processing. Trans-fatty acids occur in some margarines and many types of junk food and they are damaging to cardiovascular health. Trans-fatty acids can be spotted on food labels that state their contents of hydrogenated oils or partially hydrogenated oils.

## Good Cholesterol: HDL

In contrast to the characterization of LDL and VLDL as "bad types" of cholesterol, high density lipoprotein cholesterol (HDL) is considered a "good type" of cholesterol. In simple terms, HDL exerts an effect of drawing cholesterol into the circulating blood away from its site of deposition in arterial blood vessel walls. High density lipoprotein (HDL) has a complex function. It is responsible to some degree for returning cholesterol to the liver and it directly protects the lining of blood vessels from the deposition of smaller remnants of fat that have been digested by enzymes in the blood stream.

## Ratios of HDL to LDL

The ratio of the amounts of HDL to LDL is examined in modern medicine a reasonable measure of coronary artery disease risk. In a similar way, the ratio between HDL and total cholesterol is an important measure of the risk of heart disease. The most desirable ratio of HDL to LDL is a ratio that favors a preponderance of HDL. Ratios can be confusing. For example, looking at ratios of total cholesterol to HDL leads to a desirable ratio of less than 4.5. This ratio can be altered by raising LDL or lowering HDL, tending to push the ratio higher. In contrast, or lowering LDL and raising HDL, tends to push the ratio lower.

Most healthcare givers recommend all methods of elevating HDL to improve cardiovascular health. Exercise and moderate drinking of alcohol are associated with modest elevations of HDL. However, the recommendation of alcohol intake, even in modest amounts, is not volunteered by the healthcare giver because of the "downside" of drinking. I believe that moderate alcohol intake is safe, even accepting the oxidizing and free-radical producing effects of alcohol. However, the presence of a low HDL or high blood cholesterol cannot be used as a reason to advise people to drink. Several other conditions or factors affect blood HDL levels (Table 14).

| Decrease HDL | Increase HDL |
|---|---|
| Vegetarian Diet | Oral Estrogens, ? phytoestregens (Female sex hormones) |
| Cigarettes | Exercise |
| Sedentary Lifestyle | Alcohol (moderate intake) |
| Obesity | Lean Body Mass |
| Menopause, Androgens, Progestogens | Normal Function of Insulin |

Table 14: Conditions or agents that alter high density lipoprotein (HDL) cholesterol Levels (good cholesterol). Note: a low overall fat intake, as occurs in the presence of a strict vegan diet, lowers all types of blood lipids, including HDL. Lowering HDL is a "downside" of a vegan lifestyle.

In summary, the aims of altering blood lipids to promote

cardiovascular health are to achieve a low LDL, a low VLDL, low triglycerides, a high HDL, a low total cholesterol and HDL cholesterol ratios. Cardiovascular disease caused by atheroma (a buildup of fat and cholesterol in arterial blood vessels) is at the root of the occurrence of cardiovascular disease, the number one cause of death in Western society.

## Optimal Blood Lipid Levels?

The exact levels of blood cholesterol and other lipids that can be considered healthy for an individual cannot be determined precisely, but in May 2001, new guidelines were issued for the definition , prevention and management of high blood cholesterol. These new guidelines were proposed by the National Cholesterol Education Program in conjunction with the National Heart, Lung and Blood Institute and they redefined acceptable levels of blood fats (Table 15). The new definitions have revised down optimal blood levels of bad cholesterol (LDL and triglycerides), whilst revising good cholesterol (HDL) upwards (Table 15). Among the most significant aspects of these new recommendations was the recognition of the need to expand management to all risk factors for heart disease. Using revised definitions the number of Americans with abnormal blood lipids is estimated to be more than 100 million, compared with 65 million prior to the new guidelines.

On occasion, individuals with high blood cholesterol may live to a ripe old age without cardiovascular problems. Conversely, some with low blood cholesterol may die prematurely. The reason why the cholesterol theory is not "foolproof" explanation of cardiovascular risk is because factors other than cholesterol play a pivotal role in causing heart disease and other cardiovascular problems. Again, this reinforces the "mixed bag of dirty tricks" within Syndrome X and the concept of the "bouquet of barbed wire" of cardiovascular risk factors.

| Total Cholesterol | Desirable: Less than 200 mg/dL<br>Borderline high: 200 to 239 mg/dL<br>High: Greater than 240 mg/dL |
|---|---|
| LDL Cholesterol | Optimal: Less than 100 mg/dL<br>Near-optimal: 100 to 129 mg/dL<br>Borderline high: 130 to 159 mg/dL<br>High: 160 to 189 mg/dL<br>Very high: 190 mg/dL and greater |
| HDL Cholesterol | Low: Less than 40 mg/dL<br>Optimal: 60 mg/dL<br>High: Greater than 60 mg/dL |
| LDL to HDL Ratio | less than 4:5 |
| Triglycerides | 50 to 150 mg/dl (more aggressive controls recommended) |

**Table 15:** A Guide to the Levels of Blood Lipids. Note: These guidelines were proposed by the National Institutes of Health in May 2001. These are new targets for blood lipids which are recommended with more holistic efforts to reduce cardiovascular risks. Opinion differs in some medical circles on ideal targets for blood lipids and in the presence of heart disease controls of blood cholesterol are necessarily more stringent.

Evidence has emerged that some nutritionally based interventions may achieve optimal blood lipid (fat or cholesterol) levels and they may partially reverse established arteriosclerotic disease (hardened, clogged arteries) (see Sections 7 and 8). Recently, the importance of unstable plaque in blood vessels as a high risk for cardiovascular events has made nutraceutical interventions potentially more important in therapy. Established Syndrome X promotes phases of unstable plaque formation.

THE HIGHER THE CHOLESTEROL NUMBER THE HIGHER THE RISK

It is known that the overall average range of total blood cholesterol levels of adult Americans and Western Europeans is 210 -

225 mg/dL or higher, and statistical studies demonstrate with clarity that the death rate from coronary artery disease increases with blood cholesterol levels. When the blood cholesterol level is 240 mg/dL, the death rate from cardiovascular diseases increases four-fold above the average rate. At a blood cholesterol level of 260 mg/dL, the risk of death is about six-fold, or greater. Diabetes increases heart disease risk eight fold. Thus, the threats of the components of Syndrome X reveal themselves in a "scary" manner.

It is not just the total blood cholesterol number (count) that determines risk, it is the lipid profile and, in particular, levels of LDL (blood cholesterol members) are important. Blood cholesterol levels in affluent countries are higher than those in third world countries. It should be noted, however, that in affluent societies it is the lower socioeconomic groups that may be particularly at risk. I believe that this is because high cholesterol, high fat, low fiber, high sugar containing food is relatively cheap and abundant; largely with thanks to the fast food industry and "clever" food processing. Some citizens who are often financially disadvantaged may tend to eat greater amounts of "junk" or "fast" food. This situation is one of the reasons why some African Americans, Native North American Indians and Hispanics have real problems with Syndrome X. I wish this situation would change, quickly !

## SOCIAL, AGE, GENDER AND ETHNIC OBSERVATIONS

It has been recognized that there are certain risk factors for coronary artery disease that cannot be readily abolished. We reflect on advancing age and male gender as obvious "encumbrances". The lower prevalence of heart disease in premenopausal women (women generally less than 50 years of age) is quite striking. The incidence of coronary artery disease in women who are premenopausal is approximately equivalent to that found in men who are about 15 years younger. However, it is sometimes forgotten that coronary artery disease is the most common cause of death in women, as it is in men. There is much concern about the management of coronary artery disease in women because evidence has emerged that it may be often under-diagnosed in the female; and it may be managed sometimes in a much less assertive manner than it is in males.

It is apparent that deaths from coronary artery disease have not declined to the same degree in African Americans or Hispanics or Native Americans as they have in Caucasians. I believe that this is due to many circumstances. Certainly, poor nutrition plays a major role in this circumstance. Minority groups have much less access to education on intervention strategies to reduce the risks of cardiovascular disease. Syndrome X is a silent killer that is a successful predator among both our less privileged sector of society and our affluent sector of society. Syndrome X knows no social or ethnic boundaries. These situations must change. Whilst medical literature has focused on lower socioeconomic status and Syndrome X, there are affluent ethnic groups for whom Syndrome X is a particular problem. Dr. Elliot Goldberg MD, a physician in Israel who works primarily with Hasidic communities has commented on the emergence of diabetes, hypertension, and obesity (Syndrome X) in Hasidic Jews and he has related this to lifestyle (notably, lack of exercise).

## OBSESSION WITH BLOOD CHOLESTEROL NUMBERS: DO NOT FORGET OTHER ISSUES

It is easy to become obsessed by cholesterol numbers. Perhaps, patients and doctors place too much emphasis on the apparent "magic numbers" of blood tests. A healthy adult would ideally have a blood cholesterol in the range of 120 - 180 mg/dL. However, there is little point in having a blood cholesterol of 120 mg/dL and continuing to smoke or drink excessively. Several studies have confirmed that excessive calorie, saturated fat, cholesterol intake and salt are among the commonest nutritional threats to health in Western Society. Overall, about 60% of all Americans may have high blood cholesterol, 80% eat too much fat and/or protein and 50% take too much salt in their diet. Studies on the population's consumption of refined sugar is equally striking. The growth in world consumption of sugar has increased from 30 million tons in 1950 to more than 110 million tons in the 1990's. Average consumption of sucrose and fructose in Western populations is about 50 kg/individual (or more) which represents at least 25% of total calorie intake. The "sweetening" of America has soured its health.

Current concepts of "What constitutes a high blood cholesterol" level emanated originally from epidemiological data (population studies) on blood lipids that were collected from more than 60,000 individuals in 10 different population groups in the United States. It has been accepted by some physicians that 200 mg/dL is the maximum acceptable total cholesterol level regardless of age or sex Other more stringent definitions of "normality" stem from observations that the relationship between cholesterol levels and coronary vascular disease is a continuous-"graded"-risk rather than an artificial threshold at 200 mg/dL. Some authorities have placed the maximum acceptable total blood cholesterol level at 180 mg/dL for adults , whilst others stress 160 mg/dL.

The significance of looking at cholesterol numbers relates to their use as a measure of risk. It has been estimated that for each one percent of reduction in blood cholesterol levels, there is a two percent reduction in coronary heart disease. However, at "low levels" of blood cholesterol the advantages of going lower are not apparent. Figure 2 is a very important schematic graph that shows the relationship between blood cholesterol (bad cholesterol) and heart disease appears to be shaped like a "hockey stick". Note: At extremes of blood cholesterol levels, it is not a straight line relationship where incremental levels of bad types of blood cholesterol are related to cardiovascular disease. One must look at the ends of the "hockey stick curve" that shows the changing relationship between blood cholesterol and cardiac deaths.

---

**Syndrome X is assisted by
nutritional factors that do more than
"just" lower blood cholosterol.
(See Section 8)**

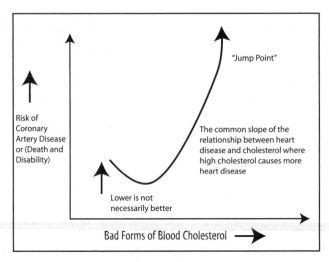

**Figure 2**: The relationship between the risk of heart disease and blood cholesterol levels is not a simple relationship. The curve looks like a "hockey stick" where at very low levels of blood cholesterol the risk of death from all causes increases and at very high levels of blood cholesterol the cardiovascular risk jumps dramatically. Provided by permission Natures Benefit Inc© (www.naturesbenefit.com)

## CHOLESTEROL TARGETS DEFINED:
## SPECIAL TARGETS FOR SPECIAL CIRCUMSTANCES

I hinted that there has been continuing argument about the optimal levels of blood cholesterol which are desirable for good health. Higher blood cholesterol levels can be perhaps tolerated in individuals who have no other significant risk factors. Currently, it is acceptable, by some, (following non-standard guidelines) for an individual to have a blood cholesterol level of up to 200 mg/dL, in the absence of any other cardiovascular risk factors. When multiple risk factors are present, it is advised that the target blood cholesterol level be less than 130 mg/dL. A significant portion of our population fall into this category and the achievement of a blood cholesterol of this level is often quite difficult for individuals faced with the temptations of adverse lifestyle in Western society.

## Shooting for the Lowest Cholesterol Number

The benefits of aggressive lowering of blood cholesterol in patients with coronary artery disease are much clearer than they are in otherwise healthy people. It is advisable for a person with established coronary artery disease to "shoot for the lowest cholesterol level possible" and the optimal target may be less than 100 mg/dL! The person with coronary artery disease is advised to try and get the blood HDL level to above 35 mg/dL. Individuals with established coronary artery disease should be quite diligent about strategies to elevate blood HDL levels, but I stress that achieving this situation can often be quite difficult.

In recent years, medical scientists have discovered that people with very low cholesterol may not be as healthy as anticipated (Figure 2). This circumstance is explained in many ways but essentially these findings are used to question the value of very low cholesterol levels, except in people with heart disease. The problem is that lowering cholesterol in the diet tends to result in the lowering of both LDL and HDL cholesterol. The undesirable reduction in HDL could be amenable to the incorporation of soluble fiber or certain fractions of soluble fiber (and perhaps soy protein or fish oil) into the diet, because some elevation of HDL is recorded in patients taking diets enriched with these substances (see Section 7: The Secret of Soluble Fiber and "The Soy Revolution," Holt S., Dell Inc.)

## Pivotal Studies Linking Cholesterol and Coronary Artery Disease

Coincidental with the political statements in the early 1950's that Western populations "had never had it so good" was the initiation of the Framingham Study, by the National Institute of Health. It is ironic that "never having it so good" was linked clearly with coronary heart disease in the Framingham Study. The era of new found prosperity in Western Europe and the U.S. following the second world war may have been responsible for a significant proportion of the recent illnesses and deaths from cardiovascular disease.

So strong was the association of high blood cholesterol and

coronary artery disease in the Framingham Study, that Dr. W.P. Castelli and his associates were able to publish a classic scientific paper in 1983 titled "Summary Estimates of Cholesterol Used to Predict Coronary Heart Disease". This study was very valuable but its "literal interpretation" as a "gospel" did much to skew ideas to the singular importance of high blood cholesterol in the causation of heart disease. The Framingham Study is an example of one of the most complete and longest prospective studies of lifestyle as a cause of coronary heart disease, and stroke. The data from this study characterized the heart attack victim to have an average blood cholesterol of 244 mg% with a range of 220-260 mg%.

Several other studies clearly relate high blood cholesterol to coronary artery disease. Of importance are the Oslo Study and the Zutphen Study that provide evidence that coronary artery disease can be prevented to some degree by lowering a high blood cholesterol. The Oslo Study, in Norway, examined 1,234 mature males who were split into two groups. One group modified its diet and adverse lifestyle with an emphasis on lowering blood cholesterol, whereas the other group formed a control group and received no such interventions. After five years, the incidence of heart attacks was 47% lower in the group with the lifestyle and dietary interventions compared with the control group.

The Zutphen Study, in Holland, lasted 20 years during which 852 middle-aged males had their diets and lifestyles assessed prior to entering a prospective study of the development of coronary artery disease. This study showed a cardio-protective effect of the incorporation of dietary fiber and fish (fish oil) in the diet and further defined adverse lifestyle as a determinant of coronary deaths and disability (see later Sections 7 and 8 in this book).

A consideration of the Framingham, Oslo, and Zutphen studies underscores the importance of blood cholesterol reduction and correction of adverse lifestyle in the prevention of coronary artery disease. Modern science identifies some individuals at risk where the "writing is one the wall" in terms of poor cardiovascular health. Table 15 summarizes the characteristics of individuals who are best advised to take immediate corrective action to reduce their risk of coronary heart disease.

- Individuals with insulin resistance, glucose intolerance or diabetes mellitus
- Adult smokers
- Women experiencing the climacteric (menopause)
- Hypertensive females or males, especially over the age of 30 (sustained BP > 140/80mmHg)
- Mature men and women over the age of 50 years
- Individuals who are more than fifteen pounds above average body weight
- Hypercholesterolemia in the adult.
- Women taking the contraceptive pill?
- Individuals with Type A behavior
- Victims of "lousy lifestyle"

**Table 15:** Characteristics of individuals who are advised to consider early measures to reduce cardiovascular risks. This list is not complete. It represents a different way of "spelling out" a combat against Syndrome X and the "bouquet of barbed wire".

## WHEN THE TREATMENT IS WORSE THAN THE DISEASE

Iatrogenic (healthcare induced) disease is rampant. When the safety of medical treatments go out of the window, alternative medicine is invited through the door. One of the principal reasons for an individual to seek alternative medical treatments is disenchantment with standard (conventional) therapies (allopathic approaches). The last 50 years has seen an explosion in new drug development resulting in an array of drugs that are highly effective at relieving symptoms of disease, but less effective at altering the clinical course of many chronic diseases.

Modern humankind has embraced the "quick fix approach" where "popping a pill" may melt symptoms. It is well recognized that symptom relief is the number one drive to use both prescription and over the counter drugs. This temporary sense of well-being has led many people to perceive that there is a pharmaceutical cure out there for most ailments. This misguided complacency has led to a failure of many preventive medicine strategies, especially those that involve lifestyle change. Furthermore, rapid symptom relief from a drug may actually reinforce the continuation of adverse lifestyle that contributes to disease process causing the symptoms. These factors operate in the classic approach to blood cholesterol-lowering with drugs, perhaps, somewhat to the detriment of public health.

## Chapter Summary

High blood cholesterol is only one component of the bigger picture of Syndrome X and the "bouquet of barbed wire" of cardiovascular risk factors. First line options to lower blood cholesterol do not include drugs. Correcting high blood cholesterol per se is important, but the contribution of insulin resistance should be considered in corrective actions. First line approaches to lower blood cholesterol are lifestyle change and nutritional interventions, including the appropriate use of selected dietary supplements (Sections 7 and 8). Several cholesterol-lowering drugs may not be safe and they are not universally cost effective. The role of nutritional interventions in correction of the cardinal components of Syndrome X will become more obvious as we progress in our discussions.

# COMBAT DIABETES: INSULIN RESISTANCE AND GLUCOSE INTOLERANCE

## DIABETES: A SIPHON OF HEALTH

Diabetes mellitus is a common disease that is increasing in prevalence. It involves the basic lack or malfunction of the actions of insulin resulting in high blood sugar. The word "diabetes" is derived from a Greek word that means "siphon", presumably related to the ability of the high blood sugar to cause fluid loss from the body, mainly as a consequence of excessive urination. It is recorded that the scholar Aretaeus of Cappadocia coined the word diabetes two centuries ago (approximately 100 AD), but the disease may have been first noted by the Egyptian Papyrus Ebers in 1500 BC, or thereabouts. Mellitus means sweet and it typifies the taste of urine from affected individuals. Strange as it may seem, early physicians often made a diagnosis of diabetes mellitus by tasting urine.

Diabetes mellitus is a major cause of death and disability and it affects individuals of all ages. In its most common form, it is called maturity onset diabetes mellitus (or Type 2 diabetes). Type 2 diabetes is caused by a complex interplay of lifestyle factors, resistance to insulin progressing to lack of insulin and obesity.

Understanding diabetes mellitus involves a knowledge of the handling of glucose by the body and the ability of high levels of blood
sugar to "siphon" health from the body.

## GLUCOSE TOLERANCE: THE BASICS

Glucose (sugar) enters the body from the digestive tract and
it is distributed throughout the body with the help of insulin, but
other body hormones play a role. Insulin drives glucose into many
cells where it is used as fuel to supply the energy needs of the body.
Without the presence or actions of insulin, blood sugar (glucose)
will tend to rise and the body appears to be "intolerant" of glucose
(glucose intolerance). On the other hand, when insulin works effectively, glucose balance or tolerance exists. Without insulin, "glucose
intolerance" is present. When one eats carbohydrates, glucose will
tend to rise in the blood stream within certain limits. The body
keeps glucose within quite a strict range in the blood (50 mg per 100
ml of blood to 150 mg per 100 ml of blood), largely as a result of
the actions of insulin and glucagon.

One can recognize that there are normal fluctuations in
blood sugar (glucose) throughout a 24 hour period. Between meals,
other aspects of body metabolism (chemistry) control the blood
sugar levels within a close range of about 70 to 110 mg of glucose
per 100 ml of blood. One important process is the storage of sugar
in the body by the liver. Glucose is stored in this manner in a series
of "bigger" (complex) sugar molecules known as glycogen.
Glycogen is the body's store of sugar, but it is used quickly over a
variable period of time if fasting or strenuous exercise occurs. Thus,
glycogen is not a very efficient store of energy. The biggest stores
of energy are found in fats which can be broken down and used in
the form of triglycerides. Glucose can come from other sources,
including the conversion and breakdown of body proteins into
sugar. Protein breakdown occurs with prolonged fasting. This loss
of structural proteins from prolonged fasting is best avoided in
attempts to control weight. Healthy weight loss should not involve
loss of lean body mass (muscles). These facts are important in our
understanding of healthy weight loss (see Section 5, Obesity and
The Slim Chance).

## Understanding Diabetes Mellitus

Diabetes mellitus is a common disease in which excessive levels of blood glucose (sugar) occur. In simple terms, diabetes is generally due to the absence or lack of effective functioning of insulin. Two common types of diabetes are described. The first type (Type 1 diabetes mellitus) has been called "juvenile onset diabetes" where there is damage to the cells in the pancreas that secrete insulin. This type of diabetes occurs from a lack or absence of insulin and it tends to occur in young people, as the name suggests.

The second, but main type of diabetes (Type 2 diabetes), is commonly called "maturity onset diabetes" (MOD). Type 2 diabetes is much more common than Type 1 diabetes and it accounts for more than 90% of all known cases of diabetes. This type of diabetes is often associated in its early phases with a resistance to insulin. Insulin may be present in early forms of Type 2 diabetes, but it is not able to do its job of driving glucose into cells. Type 2 diabetes is the type of diabetes that is most relevant to our understanding of the abnormalities of body chemistry (metabolic disturbances) that cause Syndrome X. Whilst maturity onset (Type 2) diabetes occurs most often in mature people, a striking increase occurrence in this type of diabetes in children has been experienced in recent years. This disorder has been called maturity onset diabetes of the young (MODY), a strange label!

Whilst there are at least two distinct types of diabetes (Type 1 and Type 2) each type can cause similar medical complications. These complications are due to elevated blood sugar which is common to both types of diabetes; and they include cardiovascular disease, nerve damage (neuropathy), eye disease (retinopathy) and kidney disorders. Whilst much of our discussion will address Type 2 diabetes (maturity onset or maturity onset type of diabetes in young people), one cannot completely separate Type 1 and Type 2 diabetes and some overlap exists between these disorders. There is a third type of diabetes called Gestational Diabetes that occurs somewhat temporarily in pregnancy. Gestational Diabetes involves insulin resistance and research has characterized it to have much in common with Syndrome X. Diabetes is a heterogeneous disease.

## A Short Overview of Diabetes

In the disease Diabetes Mellitus the body does not produce enough insulin or the body does not respond to insulin (insulin resistance). Common symptoms in type 2 diabetes include:

- **Constant thirst and/or hunger**
- **Frequent Urination**
- **Blurred vision**
- **Lack of energy**
- **Weight loss** (or Yo Yo weight)

A characteristic of Type 2 diabetes is its association with obesity, hypertension, high blood cholesterol and early heart disease (the killer combination of Syndrome X). Our "Westernized lifestyle" seems to be a major cause of Syndrome X and insulin resistance is a fundamental problem in Syndrome X and it is a fore-runner to Type 2 diabetes mellitus. The American Diabetes Association makes it very clear that the goals of treatment of Type 2 diabetes involve:

- **Meal planning with nutritional intervention**
- **Exercise**
- **Weight Loss**
- **Drugs as a "back up plan"**

Recent scientific studies performed at Harvard University and the National Institutes of Health show that diabetes (Type 2) is preventable by moderate, weight loss and exercise.

## The Failure to Respond to Insulin's Command

Type 2 diabetes may often evolve from insulin resistance, where the command of insulin is not heeded by body tissues. Insulin resistance is the key to understanding of the progressive problems that occur in Syndrome X. When the body tissues do not respond to insulins' commands, the pancreas starts to secrete more insulin, but this occurs to no avail, at least in terms of balancing blood glucose. Excessive circulating blood insulin is not a healthy state for the body as it tends to cause increases in fat storage, cholesterol production and blood pressure. These changes result in damage to blood vessels (causing microvascular disease and clogged blood vessels, atheroma). Thus, the chain of events in Syndrome X appears to be largely triggered by insulin resistance which causes compensatory insulin excess and unwanted change in body functions (metabolic disturbances of Syndrome X or the "metabolic syndrome").

Our knowledge of the adverse results of excessive insulin makes an understanding of the causes of insulin resistance very important. Although the precise reasons why insulin resistance occurs are not known, insulin resistance tends to run in families (hereditary or genetic component) and it is made worse or precipitated by adverse lifestyle habits. These habits are well recognized in modern society and they include lack of exercise, poor diet with nutritional deficiencies and substance abuse (smoking and drinking). Of particular importance may be excessive intake of simple sugars in our diet which tend to cause excessive insulin secretion. Elegant research has confirmed that a multitude of lifestyle issues make Syndrome X and Type 2 diabetes worse. Thus, interventions that control these damaging factors can improve Type 2 diabetes and Syndrome X, or even eliminate the problems.

## ROLLERCOASTER BLOOD SUGAR

The body has clever controls over blood sugar. When blood sugar falls, a condition called hypoglycemia (hypo=low, glycemia=blood sugar) occurs. The body has very efficient ways to correct low blood sugar, especially by using hormones. Several hormones work in an opposite manner to insulin. These hormones (glucagon, cortisol, epinephrine, norepinephrine and growth hormone) will tend to cause blood sugar to rise. Whilst an appreciation of all the intricacies of blood sugar control is difficult to understand for individuals without medical training, it is more simple to consider what happens in general terms. Hormones can act to make the liver release glucose (glucagon) and stress hormones (cortisol, epinephrine etc.) act to raise blood glucose levels (see discussions on hypoglycemia, later in this chapter).

When blood sugar gets too high (greater than 150 mg%), it

spills into the urine through the kidneys. This situation leads to a loss of many body chemicals including water, minerals and vitamins, especially vitamin C and those of the B complex. Thus, repeated elevations of blood sugar place a repeated drain on vital body nutrients which can predispose an individual to many problems including impaired cardiovascular, respiratory and immune function. In addition, high blood sugar itself is damaging to tissues and it contributes to eye, kidney and nervous system complications of diabetes. I believe that many people with diabetes mellitus may benefit from balanced vitamin and mineral supplement intake.

## ACTIONS OF INSULIN

Insulin can be viewed as a hormone that plays a major role in distributing glucose throughout the body. Glucose is fuel for the chemistry of the body and it provides energy to support the chemistry of life. When blood glucose increases after a meal, insulin is secreted by special cells in the pancreas gland (Islets of Langerhans) and it acts to channel glucose into cells where it can be consumed as energy or stored as glycogen (in the liver) or fat in the organs and around the general framework of the body. During times of fasting the body can derive energy from other sources including glucose from the liver breakdown of glycogen, triglycerides from fat, and amino acids (protein) from body structures such as muscles. A limited source of energy for the body may come from acids or ketones in states of starvation or untreated diabetes. This is an unhealthy status of the body called "ketosis". It is clear that in states of health, insulin controls body functions with exquisite precision and harmony. In contrast, insulin resistance leads to Syndrome X (and the status of Syndrome X, Y and Z…).

Table 16 illustrates the many factors that raise or lower blood sugar. It is notable that all of them that result in a beneficial effect involve the selection of a healthy lifestyle.

| Raising blood sugar | Lowering blood sugar |
|---|---|
| Poor lifestyle, obesity (associated with insulin resistance) | Good lifestyle, normal body weight |
| Stress (cortisol and epinephrine) | Contentment |
| Simple sugars in diet | Diets with 30-40% healthy fat, normal protein and complex carbohydrates with fiber (High glycemic index foods) |
| Low fiber diet | High fiber diet |
| Sedentary lifestyle | Exercise |
| Added illnesses e.g. fever, heart disease, injuries | Optimum health (taking care of yourself) |
| Substance abuse e.g. alcohol, smoking, certain prescription drugs (water pills etc.) | Good lifestyle |
| Nutrient deficiencies e.g. B vitamins Chromium, omega 3 fatty acids | Good macro and micronutrient intake. |

**Table 16:** Factors that can raise or lower blood sugar. Some can act by enhancing or blocking the actions of insulin. These issues are important in prevention and treatment of Syndrome X, diabetes and other conditions that determine cardiovascular risk.

## Understanding the Concepts of Syndrome X

Syndrome X has not yet piqued widespread interest in conventional medicine, but it constitutes one of the most important public health initiatives facing Western society, especially in the combat against cardiovascular disease. Insulin resistance initiates a chain of events that tend to cause changes in body chemistry which result in Syndrome X. These changes result in high blood cholesterol, damage to the linings of arterial blood vessels, a tendency to obesity and intolerance to simple carbohydrates in the diet. This combination of problems set the stage for the progression of Syndrome X and its consequences. (Syndrome X, Y, and Z. . .)

Attempts to distinguish the precise differences between Syndrome X and type 2 diabetes have created some confusion. The easiest way to understand the differences is that in Syndrome X the main issue is resistance to insulin. This resistance results in excessive insulin secretion into the blood stream (hyperinsulinemia), whereas in type 2 diabetes (maturity onset diabetes) insulin resistance may be present but the insulin secreting cells of the pancreas "quit" and not enough insulin is available to overcome the resistance to insulin. Whilst insulin resistance is of primary importance in the development of Type 2 diabetes, a defect in the function of the cells in the pancreas that secrete insulin is often present. Type 2 diabetes has a lack of insulin at the root of its cause. To look at the circumstances from a different perspective, insulin resistance and Syndrome X are sometimes stages in the development of maturity onset diabetes, but not all people with Syndrome X will necessarily develop diabetes and some may not live long enough to develop diabetes!

It has been proposed that insulin resistance triggers the disorders within Syndrome X and these disorders evolve in a progressive manner. Changes in several areas of body chemistry work together to progress to Syndrome X, but this progression is variable in its manifestations and "partial" components of Syndrome X can "pop up" without the "full blown" picture of the killer constellation of Syndrome X (Figure 1, Section 1).

To further understand this variable status of Syndrome X, one may consider that insulin resistance may wax and wane. Intermittent returns of insulin sensitivity, in the presence of high blood insulin levels, can cause occasional low blood sugar (hypoglycemia), even though the overall problems relate more to the adverse effects of high blood sugar. I believe that intermittent hypoglycemia in people with insulin resistance precipitates sugar craving which stimulates refined sugar intake that further promotes the development of Syndrome X. Perhaps the most important other issues to consider in Syndrome X are the effect of factors such as adverse lifestyle (e.g. smoking or excessive alcohol intake) and genetic makeup of the individual. Hereditary influences and poor lifestyle are known to contribute to the progression and adverse outcome of insulin resistance and Syndrome X.

## MORE ABOUT THE PROGRESSION OF SYNDROME X

In the early part of the 1980's, medical researchers set about the task of understanding how insulin resistance operated and to characterize its presence in individuals. Prior to these detailed studies, it was known that the actions of insulin varied greatly from person to person, as measured in the laboratory by the degree to which certain cells could use sugar. It was also recognized that when enough insulin could not be secreted by the pancreas to overcome insulin resistance, type 2 (maturity onset) diabetes occurred.

The most important advances in our knowledge about the evolution of Syndrome X were the ability to understand how insulin resistance (and Syndrome X) increased the risks of cardiovascular disease. In his excellent book, Dr. G Reaven and his co-authors described "seven monkey wrenches" that Syndrome X place in "our healthy heart machinery" (Syndrome X, Reaven G, Strom TK and Fox B, Simon and Schuster, NY, 2000). Table 17 summarizes Reaven's "seven monkey wrenches".

| Increased risk for heart disease | Comment |
|---|---|
| Elevated tryglycerides in blood | Excessive insulin signals to the liver to produce triglyceride rich blood fats (VLDL) |
| Low levels of high density lipoprotein cholesterol (good cholesterol) | A switch of triglycerides among blood fats lowers good types of cholesterol |

| | |
|---|---|
| Lack of efficient clearing of blood fats after a meal | After a meal containing fat, the fats in the form of chylomicrons are not cleared rapidly |
| Changes or increases in bad cholesterol (LDL) | Bad cholesterol can change its configuration (density) and become more damaging |
| Too much clot forming proteins | Fibrinogen which converts to fibrin in a clot is present in excess in Syndrome X |
| A slowdown in blood clot removing processes in the body | A rise occurs in activator sub–stances that tend to form blood clots. Clots can block arteries, especially coronary arteries, resulting in a heart attack |

**Table 17: Syndrome X elevates risks of heart disease often by elevating** bad cholesterol. The contents of this table are modified but based on the work of Dr. G Reaven, cited in text. I add that Syndrome X tends to promote the formation of "unstable plaque" in arterial blood vessels.

Whilst the results of insulin resistance or Syndrome X (Table 17) help to characterize the basis for cardiovascular risks of stroke, heart disease and other circulatory disorders, they are not the whole story. One must again revisit the issues of adverse lifestyle that make Syndrome X worse and consider the important independent risk factors of elevations of bad cholesterol and high blood homo-cysteine levels. I reiterate that poor nutrition, substance abuse, obesity and lack of exercise all operate to make Syndrome X progress and make its outcome more serious.

LIFESTYLE AND SYNDROME X

Our understanding of the global and complex nature of cardiovascular risks begins to explain why the elimination of one risk factor will not necessarily combat cardiovascular disease. Contrary to assertions by some researchers in the famous Framingham Heart Disease Studies, heart attacks do occur in people with normal levels of "good" and "bad" cholesterol, but they do occur less frequently. One illuminating observation in the Framingham Study was that insulin resistance was associated with low blood levels of HDL (good cholesterol). Furthermore, people with controlled hypertension still had heart attacks, perhaps because many of them had the residual components of multiple risks related to insulin resistance and Syndrome X or high blood levels of homocysteine.

When Dr. Reaven first described Syndrome X in 1988, he recognized that his description of this metabolic disorder was incomplete and he did not focus on the importance of obesity. Other medical researchers started to show how genetic tendencies and body habitus (fatness, aerobic fitness levels etc.) altered the ability of an individual to handle sugar in the diet (glucose tolerance). Studies in families showed a clustering of insulin resistance confirming the importance of hereditary tendencies towards Syndrome X, but genetics did not explain the whole picture. These findings may serve as a caution to new drug developments that focus too much on genomic sciences, where it has to be assumed that genes determine protein functions in the body, in an overriding manner.

Many studies have shown how adverse lifestyle can increase cardiovascular risk and, predictably, poor habits contribute variably to the initiation and progression of Syndrome X. Physical activity improves sugar utilization and works against insulin resistance. Smoking enhances resistance to insulin, as does excessive alcohol drinking and perhaps excessive intake of caffeine (cola and coffee). Of clear significance is the contribution of poor diet with excessive consumption of calories and refined carbohydrates, and the absence of "low glycemic index" foods like fiber (foods that do not cause rapid rises in blood sugar, or high glycemic index foods). Excessive salt and saturated fat intake and too much protein of animal origin all contribute to the progression of Syndrome X. Being fat (obesity) is particularly damaging because insulin resistance and obesity go "hand in hand".

Whilst some people are fed up with a sermon on lifestyle, one must recognize that lifestyle is something we can change. One cannot easily change genetic risks but one can even impact these hereditary risks favorably by adopting a healthy lifestyle. Thus, hereditary risks must not be perceived necessarily as fixed and inevitable. There are many reasons to overcome complacency and fail to accept the "fattening of America" with its associated poor lifestyle habits. I am not lacking in sensitivity, nor do I wish to single out obesity as the sole culprit. There are some "thin" people with Syndrome X. In addition, there are healthy, overweight people without Syndrome X, but we can see the wisdom of tackling all risks, in order to stay out of the "bouquet of barbed wire".

## DIET LOOMS STRONG IN THE SOLUTION

It is clear that diet plays a major role in facilitating insulin resistance and the evolution of Syndrome X. Simple sugars are consumed in Western Society in staggering amounts. These sugars "gyrate" blood sugar and test the resources of insulin controls in the body. Unfortunately, sugar comes with many positive behavioral reinforcements. It tastes good and it satisfies the cravings which are caused, in part, by insulin resistance itself! The real evil is that refined sugar may be recognized by the individual as alleviating temporarily some symptoms associated with the progression of Syndrome X, especially if hypoglycemia (low blood sugar) occurs. Anything that tends to promote insulin secretion in the presence of insulin resistance will tend to make Syndrome X gallop in its progression. We shall learn that a limitation of dietary intake of simple sugars is necessary to combat Syndrome X. Less obvious is the need to enhance our intake of healthy types of fats (especially omega 3 fatty acids) and limit animal protein intake. Certain amino acids derived from dietary protein can act to release insulin. These issues will become clearer as we develop a dietary approach to combat Syndrome X (see Sections 5, 6 and 10).

## DERIVING THE COMBAT SYNDROME X DIET

If one area of popular medicine creates confusion, it is "a diet for this" and "a diet for that". To impose a significant change on the quantity and type of food that an individual eats is a serious business which has been fraught historically with failure. Dietary adjustments must have general health as an objective, not "just" weight loss, "just" lowering cholesterol etc. The effect of the "combat Syndrome X Diet" is to go to the very basis of the problem – most notably insulin resistance. It is the release and actions of insulin that do the damage.

One must have good reasons to reject diets that are proposed by The American Heart Association (AHA), The American Diabetes Association  ADA, The National Cholesterol Education Program, The USDA and even those presented by diet gurus e.g. The Atkins Diet, The Zone Diet, Sugarbusters and The Carbohydrate Addicts Diet etc. There has never been a time in medicine where such mass confusion prevails on a common health initiative such as a "good diet". The whole situation can be rationalized by stating emphatically that there is no single, ideal dietary approach that is portable to everyone's perceived need or everyone's objective of "one diet for health". Diets are like well-fitting clothes, they are tailored to the individuals' needs.

Before, I precipitate disappointment by not giving a magic solution to the "diet issue", dietary approaches are quite simple if the needs of an individual are well characterized.  The features of the combat Syndrome X diet are summarized as:

1) **The diet must be part of a plan to alter adverse lifestyle e.g. exercise, avoidance of substance abuse.**
2) **The diet must be applied with modification of eating behavior – essentially a lifestyle issue.**
3) **The diet must be designed to address the consequences of the release and actions of insulin.**
4) **The diet must provide the vital nutrients in balanced amounts to support body structures and functions.**

To focus on the key issue of diet composition, we need to go back to basics. High carbohydrate diets, especially those incorporating refined sugars are clearly a problem in Syndrome X, because sugars release insulin. The USDA Food Pyramid and recommendations of the AHA have tended to encourage a high carbohydrate approach. Excessive protein in the diet can stress body systems and protein releases insulin, contrary to popular belief. In this regard, the Zone Diet and the Protein Power Diet do not fit completely the needs of the Combat Syndrome X plan.

Of greatest confusion is the role of fat in the diet. Fat is generally considered bad for health, but this is not necessarily the case. Whilst bad fat is "saturated" (solid) fat, good fat is unsaturated (liquid) fat. The real importance of fat is that it is very high in calories but it does not release insulin. Dietary advice to engage in liberal fat intake, even of the saturated type, is not good advice. Whilst I believe that "benign dietary ketosis" may cause appetite suppression and weight loss, I object to the use of the term "benign" and protracted ketosis is not healthy. This approach has been popularized as The Atkin's Diet (described by William Banting in the 19th Century), but it is not a good approach for Syndrome X, Y and Z...

Clearly, I am involved in basic discussions and the issues are more complex than I am able to address in simplified advice. In brief, the Combat Syndrome X diet is higher in healthy types of fat (unsaturated, especially omega 3 fatty acids), adequate in carbohydrates of the complex type (avoiding simple sugars) and adequate in protein. The adjustable Combat Syndrome X Diet is 40-45% carbohydrate (fiber and associated complex carbohydrates preferred) 35-40% fat (with a choice of healthy fat) and 15-20% protein (with a preference for the incorporation of vegetable protein, e.g. soy protein). My recommendations are not novel or new, but they do not fit current conventional medical thoughts.

I see little controversy in the recommendations that I make to address insulin release and actions by balancing calorie intake from refined sugar, but my belief that dietary supplements may often be required to address the problems of Syndrome X may raise the eyebrows of the medical establishment. In later sections of this book, I describe the powerful actions of several natural substances which may be of pivotal importance in reversing Syndrome X. These nutraceuticals (dietary supplements) include combinations of soluble fiber, extracts of soluble fiber, fatty acids from fish oil (omega-3 fatty acids) and vegetable protein (e.g. soy).

## The Dangers of Diabetes Mellitus

The individual with maturity onset diabetes, whether young or old, is often overweight and invariably has abnormal blood lipids. This situation is intimately related to Syndrome X. Weight loss alone can help prevent and even reverse diabetes mellitus and strict lifestyle changes with dietary modifications can be adequate; and sometimes it affords complete treatment for some people with maturity onset diabetes. In the past couple of decades, much evidence has emerged that the careful control of high blood glucose levels in diabetes will result in a reduction of the complications of diabetes mellitus. These "diabetic" complications include diseases of blood vessels. These blood vessel disorders of blood vessels are found in diabetes mellitus are found in small blood vessels (microvasculature) and they can cause retinopathy (eye disease), heart disease and diseases of the kidneys. Diabetes is a major cause of renal failure, i.e. kidney disease that impairs renal (kidney) function.

## INSULIN IS A FRIED AND A FOE

We recognize that insulin is necessary for blood glucose control, but it has other beneficial complex actions on the body. However, in Syndrome X it is proposed that, high levels of circulating insulin, as a consequence of insulin resistance, may tend to cause atheroma in blood vessels and other metabolic problems. It is well recognized that the phenomenon of insulin resistance is a key feature in Syndrome X The benefit of precise control of blood glucose in the reduction of arteriosclerosis affecting large or medium sized arterial vessels (blocking and hardening of arteries) is now apparent. The diabetic individual usually has multiple risk factors, including abnormalities of blood lipids and high blood pressure. These individuals can invariably exhibit the features of Syndrome X with variable severity. Aggressive control of all risk factors is very important in the management of diabetes mellitus because patients with diabetes are at special risk for the development of cardiovascular disease and other diseases.

## CONTROL OF BLOOD GLUCOSE
## REDUCES COMPLICATIONS AND DEATHS

The advantages of tight control of blood sugar in both Type 1 and Type 2 diabetes mellitus is apparent in many studies. Recent scientific literature confirms the benefits of good control of blood sugar in the prevention of complications in people with type 2 diabetes. In the United Kingdom, The Diabetes Control and Complications Trial, and the UK Prospective Diabetes Study, report a good relationship between measures of blood glucose control and diminution in health risks of individuals with maturity onset diabetes (Stratton IM, Adler AI, Neil HA and colleagues, British Medical Journal, 321, 405-12, 2000).

When the blood test Hemoglobin A1c (average measure of blood sugar control, over about 3 months) is reduced by 1%, a 21% reduction in risk of death from diabetes mellitus occurs. Furthermore, this 1% fall in Hemoglobin A!c causes a 14% reduction in risk of heart attack and a 37% reduction in microvascular disease (blood vessel disease) that causes retinopathy and other disorders. The clear message is that strict control of blood glucose reduces the risk of complications of diabetes.

## EXERCISE, DIABETES AND CORONARY RISKS

Exercise has measurable benefits in diabetes mellitus. It is well documented that individuals who have a sedentary lifestyle also have a predisposition to coronary artery disease (obesity and other features of Syndrome X). This finding is related to the fact that people who do not engage in physical activity tend to be overweight, have high blood pressure, and/or high blood cholesterol and they develop diabetes mellitus more often. Thus, enhancement of physical activity has been demonstrated in many studies to reduce the risk of coronary artery disease. Exercise is a fundamental way to combat both diabetes and other disorders within Syndrome X.

Exercise programs that can be undertaken in patients who have survived a heart attack have been shown to improve prognosis. Furthermore, physical training techniques in subjects with established coronary artery disease can be shown to reduce the incidence of death due to coronary artery disease by about 20%. However, exercise programs must be supervised in the presence of heart disease or other significant disorders. The National Diabetes Prevention Program has stressed the role of exercise in preventing maturity onset of diabetes mellitus. It seems likely that physical activity will exert a beneficial effect on all risk factors for coronary artery disease, including obesity, high blood pressure and abnormal blood lipids. However, it is surprising that relatively few controlled clinical studies have been performed in these areas of intervention. This circumstance contrasts with the thousands of clinical trials that have been undertaken to show the variable effectiveness of cholesterol-lowering drugs or anti-diabetic medications.

## Drugs for Type 2 Diabetes

The drug treatment of maturity onset diabetes is valuable, if used appropriately. I stress the qualification of "appropriate use" and echo the opinion of the American Diabetes Association that drugs are the "back up plan" for Type 2 diabetes. Most drugs used in the treatment of Type 2 diabetes work by increasing insulin production, a circumstance that may not be beneficial in the presence of insulin resistance in Syndrome X, where excess circulating insulin in the blood (hyperinsulinism) is believed to be damaging. There are drugs that work by enhancing glucose uptake by cells (e.g. biguanides). Thiazolidinediones, a relatively new class of drugs that enhance sensitivity to insulin, have been developed (e.g. rosiglitazone and pioglitazone). The idea being that with the use of thiazolidinediones the body can utilize its own insulin more efficiently.

Table 18 lists the main classes of drugs used in the treatment of Type 2 diabetes. Their use is not always cost effective and I believe that there has been a tendency to prescribe many of these drugs without exercising the first line options of lifestyle change and nutritional interventions, including the use of dietary supplements (e.g. soluble fiber or beta glucan extracts of soluble oat fiber, omega-3 fatty acids and fractions of soy). The list of side effects associated with the use of these drugs is very long and they include common adverse symptoms of a general type, sensitivity reactions, liver problems, hypoglycemia, severe disturbances of body chemistry and occasional deaths. The drug treatment of Type 2 diabetes requires close monitoring because of the common occurrence of adverse drug events.

| Drug Type | Brand/Generic Names |
|---|---|
| **Thiazolidinediones**<br>Reduce the body's resistance to its own natural insulin | Avandia® (rosiglitazone maleate)<br>Actos® (pioglitazone HCl) |

**Sulfonylureas**
Lower blood glucose
levels by pushing the pancreas
to produce and release
more insulin

Amaryl® (glimepiride tablets)
Diasseta® (glyburide)
Diabinese® (chlorpropamide)
Glucotrol® (glipizide)
Glucotrol XL® (glipizide
Glynase® PresTab® Tablets
(micronized glyburide tablets)
Micronase® Tablets (glyburide)

**Alpha-Glucosidase Inhibitors**
Slow the breakdown of
food into glucose, causing
glucose to enter the blood
more slowly

Precose® (acarbose tablets)
Glyset™ (miglitol)

**Biguanides**
Multiple ways that the drugs work;
slow the liver's release of
stored glucose,
increase glucose uptake

Glucophage® (metformin
hydrochloride tablets)
Glucophage XR™ (metformin
hydrochloride extended-release
tablets)

**Other Insulin Secretagogues**
Stimulate the pancreas to
secrete insulin

Prandin™ (repaglinide)
(i.e. Meglitinides).
Starliz™ (nateglinide)

**Biguanide & Sulfonylurea**

Glucovance™ (glyburide and
metformin HCl)

**Table 18:** Drugs that are used in the treatment of type 2 diabetes. Each class of drug possesses disadvantages or limitations. Thiazolidinediones that enhance the sensitivity of the body to insulin have a tendency to cause weight gain and liver problems. One of this group was removed due to serious liver toxicity with a tendency to raise blood cholesterol and body weight. Sulfonylureas stimulate insulin production which may be best avoided in the state of hyperinsulinism and insulin resistance. They may cause weight gain and hypoglycemia. Biguanides are old fashioned drugs with common gastrointestinal side effects and uncommon but life-threatening occurrence of lactic acidosis. Fixed combinations of Biguanides and Sulfonylureas are not able to be individually tailored to a patient's need.

Drugs are best considered the "back-up" plan for the management of maturity onset diabetes and they are generally not indicated in maturity onset diabetes occurring in young people (MODY).

## HYPOGLYCEMIA: CONTRARIAN CONCEPTS

Discussions of diabetes mellitus tend to concentrate logically on elevations of blood glucose (hyperglycemia), but the contrarian perspective of hypoglycemia (low blood sugar) is sometimes present in the course of the development of Type 2 diabetes. Whilst insulin resistance and glucose intolerance is the hallmark of Syndrome X, the occurrence of intermittent hypoglycemia as a component of this disorder may have been overlooked. Standard medical textbooks mention hypoglycemia as a minor symptom of Type 2 diabetes (or a prediabetic state) and attribute it, with caution, to the developing diabetic status itself. How does hypoglycemia (low blood sugar) happen in a disease characterized by hyperglycemia (high blood sugar)?

At first sight, insulin resistance (or lack in established Type 2 diabetes) would be expected to be consistently associated with a tendency to high blood sugar, but this consistency is not present because of the variability in the insulin resistance itself, as well as the gross variation in the amount of insulin secreted (or glucose intake that causes insulin secretion) in the developing or established circumstance of Type 2 diabetes. Insulin actions on tissue receptors can change quite dramatically in some situations. In other words, the conpensatory hyperinsulinism seen in Syndrome X (or pre-diabetes) can work to achieve a lowering of blood glucose in a variable manner and "overshoots" in the action of insulin may cause low blood sugar (hypoglycemia). Perhaps, the circumstance of blood sugar control is better perceived as a variability in insulin response, even in normal people. The variability of response has an even greater variability of response when the basic mechanisms for balancing blood glucose are disturbed e.g. in Syndrome X or anything than alters blood glucose control such as distorted eating or even exercise.

Hypoglycemia (low blood sugar) has many causes ranging from hereditary disorders to cancer (insulinoma, sarcoma) to reactive or idiopathic (unknown) circumstances. When blood sugar falls below critical levels, symptoms and signs of the "fright and flight" reaction of the body emerge due to stimulation of parts of the nervous system called the sympathetic nervous system. The sympathetic nervous system "kicks in" to try and raise the blood sugar. These events explain the symptoms of hypoglycemia such as sweating, nervousness, tremor, fainting, heart palpitations and "hunger". The hunger caused by hypoglycemia, that sometimes occurs in the individual with Syndrome X, can cause "sugar craving" which may remove the unpleasant symptom of craving, but eating sugar makes Syndrome X worse. This is a vicious cycle caused by low blood sugar in some people with Syndrome X and it operates with negative consequences, perhaps more often than we realize.

The second pattern of symptoms encountered in states of low blood sugar result from lack of glucose supply to the brain and nervous system. This situation in hypoglycemia results in episodic confusion, strange behavior (sometimes like "drunkenness"), visual disturbances and rarely seizures or loss of consciousness. In general, the central nervous system manifestations of hypoglycemia only usually occur in cases of profound lowering of blood sugar. It is interesting to note that some distinguished psychiatrists have attributed a variety of mental illnesses to undiagnosed "reactive hypoglycemia".

The term "reactive hypoglycemia" refers mainly to low blood sugar provoked by eating where insulin "overshoots" in its actions. Indeed, the occurrence of reactive hypoglycemia is the reason given for episodes of low blood glucose encountered in early cases of Type 2 diabetes (Syndrome X). I believe that this explanation is flawed and hypoglycemia of a non-reactive type is also encountered in the evolving status of Type 2 diabetes mellitus.

HYPOGLYCEMIA TODAY, DIABETES TOMORROW

In the 1970's, popular books on the contribution of hypoglycemia to a wide variety of diseases made hypoglycemia a popular self-diagnosis, but the importance of this disorder has receded in recent times. I have no doubt that hypoglycemia has been overdiagnosed, especially by the alternative medical profession in the past, but its significance should not be minimized. In order to diagnose "hypoglycemia" some physicians have used extended glucose tolerance tests where the blood sugar response to a glucose drink is measured over hours (at least 5 hours) and an interpretation is given on the extended blood glucose response. Conventional medicine rejects this practice.

Practitioners of conventional medicine have reacted against the extended oral glucose tolerance test by indicating that it results in the erroneous diagnosis of "reactive hypoglycemia", especially due to alimentary causes. Who is right? The answer I believe is that neither party is "right" or "wrong", the way of knowing how significant the control of blood sugar may be probably rests in the continuous monitoring of blood glucose over long periods of time and relating the changes in blood glucose to day to day activity and blood insulin levels (or other hormones e.g. glucagon). To get a clear picture of events, the levels of insulin that are secreted in response to changes in blood glucose should be measured at the same time. Whilst these issues are relevant to research, they explain my concept of the variability of the controls of blood sugar that are impacted by the variability of other factors. Furthermore, other hormones are involved in blood sugar control and the general status of body chemistry itself.

The significance of low blood sugar as a cause of many symptoms and its role in the progression of Type 2 diabetes mellitus were first suggested eighty years ago. In 1924, Dr. Seale Harris published a paper on the significance of hypoglycemia in the Journal of the American Medicial Association and he stressed the concept that "the low blood sugar of today is the diabetes of tomorrow" (cited by the late Carlton Fredericks in his book "Low Blood Sugar and You", Grosset and Dunlap, Publishers, NY, NY, 1969). For a period of time, physicians referred to a disorder called "Seale-Harris-Type Hypoglycemia" and I believe that this entity is waiting to be rediscovered in people with Syndrome X, especially when ambulatory monitoring of blood sugar and insulin becomes a common tool of medical investigation.

## A PANOPLY OF HORMONES

It is not possible to review all of the exciting new developments in the study of the many hormones that are involved in Syndrome X and the explanation of the linkage between obesity, insulin resistance and diabetes. It is known that about 80% of individuals with type 2 diabetes mellitus have obesity or are overweight to a variable degree. Recent scientific studies have led to the identification of a new hormone that is secreted by fat cells called "resistin" (Steppan CM and colleagues, Nature, 409, 307-312, 2001). The actions of resistin seem to explain a clear relationship between obesity and the development of type 2 diabetes. Studies in mice show that fat cells secrete resistin which is a unique signaling substance that causes a resistance to the actions of insulin and promotes glucose intolerance. The insulin sensitizing drugs (e.g. rosiglitazone) seem to act, in part, by decreasing levels of resistin in obese mice that have dietary induced or hereditary forms of obesity. Perhaps resistin is a key in the chain of events in Syndrome X and this hormone seems to link obesity and type 2 diabetes together.

Much further research is required before resistin can be assumed to explain some of the missing links between obesity and diabetes. Other explanations of the link include higher levels of fatty acids in obese individuals and the secretion of many other molecules or hormones from fat tissue including tumor necrosis factor-alpha (TNF-alpha) and leptin, but these factors have not formed a complete explanation of the obesity-diabetes link. The importance of the hormone leptin in weight control has not been completely verified in humans, even though its function in animals seemed quite clear in early research. Drugs or molecules can be made to combat these hormonal mechanisms that link obesity and diabetes. As the genetic factors that cause these events become clearer, studies of the human genome will permit drug development to target key proteins that exert effects in Syndrome X and its related disorders. However, it must be remembered that it is not only hereditary factors that determine the occurrence of Syndrome X and tailored drugs developed by pharmaceutical biotechnology may be a decade away in terms of their discovery and development

NOVEL THOUGHTS ABOUT EVOLUTION AND SYNDROME X

Geneticists have hypothesized in evolutionary terms why type 2 diabetes mellitus has dramatically increased in occurrence. One of the most intriguing suggestions was made by Dr. JV Neel MD in 1962 with a description of a "thrifty" set of genes (hereditary factors) that existed in humans, but became detrimental when diets changed and became excessive in refined foods (Neel JV, Am. J. Human Genetics, 14, 353-62, 1962). This hypothesis was called "the thrifty genotype hypothesis" which basically indicated that many people had a genetic program that would render them able to store food as fat during times of abundant food supply. This kind of thrifty metabolic tendency exists in many animals e.g. bears who hibernate for the winter.

These proposals are quite interesting and may explain, in part, why certain ethnic groups are particularly prone to type 2 diabetes and Syndrome X. In fact, there is a lot of evidence that certain populations of the pacific area (Micronesians and Polynesians), American Indians and Australian Aborigines have a clear hereditary tendency to develop maturity onset diabetes. When these individuals change their lifestyle by reducing physical activity, enhancing refined sugar intake and they engage other dietary changes their thrifty genes work to their detriment and Syndrome X emerges. In other words, the evolved thrifty adjustments to famine in these populations become a major disadvantage when the excesses of current Western lifestyle are experienced by these people. America has been described as engaged in "nutritional colonialism" - notably fast food export to many third world countries, where thrifty genes operate!

Extensions of these thoughts have been applied to the habits of our distant ancestors by making much of the differences between a Paleolithic diet and a modern diet rich in refined carbohydrates and low in fiber. How relevant a study of cavemens' diets are in the explanation of Syndrome X involves a leap of logic beyond the proposals of Dr. JV Neel, but interested parties are referred to the work of Dr. S B Eaton and colleagues in the book "The Paleolithic Prescription", Harper and Row, NY, 1988.

## Different Kinds of Simple Sugars

The dietary intake of simple sugars has increased dramatically in this century and it has favored the inclusion of sucrose (table sugar) and more recently fructose. The average dietary consumption of sucrose and fructose in industrialized nations is reasonably stable at a level of 50 or more kilograms per individual, approximating to about 25 to 30% of total calorie intake in the diet. Many studies imply that this high intake of simple sugars has caused the problems found in Syndrome X, Y and Z... including hyperlipidemia, insulin resistance, hypertension, diabetic-like tissue lesions, behavioral changes, decreased fertility, and increased mortality (at least in animals). In recent times, the amount of fructose taken in the diet has increased as a consequence of the frequent use of corn syrup as a sweetener in food and beverage. Corn syrup is preferred by many food manufacturers because it is cheaper than sucrose.

Fructose is handled chemically in the body in a series of metabolic pathways that are different than those used for the handling of glucose. Fructose is metabolized largely by the liver. Like sucrose, fructose causes an increase in the activity of many body enzymes that burn sugars and promote fat storage from sugar (lipogenic activity). Fructose causes the liver to increase fat production and it may promote high blood cholesterol in the same way as glucose and sucrose. Fructose has been proposed as a more favorable type of sugar for diabetics, but this is in question. Excessive dietary intake of fructose should probably be considered a risk factor for the development of Syndrome X and especially hyperlipidemia (high blood cholesterol), as a consequence of its direct effect on fat production (lipogenesis).

Fructose may have some benefits when it is used cautiously because it may not cause overstimulation of the pancreas to produce insulin to the same degree as glucose from sucrose. In addition, fructose is known to be at least two times more sweet than glucose and it may help to reduce calorie intake in some people with exaggerated sweet-taste preferences. Furthermore, it may be better for dental health than other types of simple sugars. Much more research is required to define the negative and positive consequences of fructose intake, especially in individuals with Syndrome X. Overall, excess fructose in the diet of an individual with Syndrome X may be as damaging as excess sucrose intake.

## Protein Handling in the Presence of Diabetes Mellitus

There has been a tendency to characterize the alterations of glucose and fat metabolism by the body in the presence of diabetes mellitus, at the expense of recognizing the presence of abnormalities of protein metabolism. At the turn of the 20th century, scientists observed an increase in sugar excretion in the urine in some people with diabetes as a consequence of increased intake of protein in the diet. There has been scientific evidence, present for more than 50 years, that shows insulin to be an important regulator of the body's response to protein handling (metabolism) in relationship to general nutrient intake, with a tendency for insulin to cause retention of protein by the body. In simple terms, diabetes mellitus (insulin lack) may tend to cause a net protein loss from the body.

The recognition of abnormal protein metabolism in diabetes mellitus has led to expressed concerns about the optimum level of protein intake in the diet of people with diabetes mellitus. Recommendations have ranged from high intake to low intake and there are different protein intake recommendations for type I and type II diabetes. For example, some studies have shown that protein restriction in type I diabetes mellitus with renal complications of diabetes resulted in significant further compromise of protein metabolism and kidney function.

In common with many problems in diabetes mellitus and Syndrome X, good control of blood glucose can have a secondary, beneficial effect on protein metabolism. There has been a tendency to believe that glucose and fat metabolism are most affected by insulin, but this circumstance has undergone a reappraisal as alterations in protein handling by the body become well-described in people with diabetes. Overall, an optimal control of blood sugar in the individual with diabetes or pre-diabetes (or Syndrome X), together with a dietary intake of protein of no more than 0.8 grams per kilogram of body weight seems to be generally advisable in the presence of diabetes, but circumstances exist where different amounts of dietary protein may be required. The important effects of diabetes and insulin resistance on protein handling by the body must be considered a reason to be cautious about the use of very high protein diets or belief in "zones," created by a move to increase dietary protein intake.

## Some Lateral Thoughts (For the "Technically Inclined")

Understanding the normal and abnormal function of any endocrine organ is the cornerstone of endocrinology. The underactivity and overactivity of endocrine glands are classic principals of dichotomous thought in medicine. When it comes to diabetes mellitus, the focus of medicine has been the study of the underactivity of the Islets of Langerhans in the pancreas which secrete insulin and glucagon. Who said that the endocrine portion of the pancreas cannot be overactive? – a status of "hyperpancreatic-endocrine-function".

I believe that the relationship between symptoms experienced by individuals with Syndrome X or Type 2 diabetes mellitus may be mismatched with prevailing blood glucose levels. Temporary hyperglycemia causes few symptoms but temporary, significant hypoglycemia is always manifest. There is great inter-individual variation in the tolerance of high blood glucose or low blood glucose. Whilst one can assume that the blood glucose level per se affects the occurrence of the symptoms and signs of Syndrome X or diabetes, this may not always be the case. Furthermore, altered biochemistry as a consequence of insulin resistance in Syndrome X has variable expression. For example, the rate at which blood glucose rises or falls may be more relevant in the clinical or chemical expression of Type 2 diabetes or Syndrome X. Rapid swings of blood glucose certainly test the homeostatic powers of the insulin axis and its affiliate controls of blood glucose. This makes any incoordinate glucose-insulin responses more unpredictable and lacking in synergy ("dys-synergy").

The relevance of of the variability in all body responses that control blood glucose is illustrated by the concept of the reciprocal harmony of the body (Claude Bernard). This harmony is disturbed in Syndrome X. Anything that smoothes out the "variable variability" is desirable and this is how we can start to see the potential benefits of natural approaches e.g. beta glucan fibers smoothing out blood glucose, omega 3 fatty acids enhancing insulin sensitiv-ity etc. Picking a focussed approach with a specific drug action at one point in the disturbance of reciprocal harmony of the glucose/insulin balance is likely to have disadvantages or limitations and it may create problems.


## CHAPTER SUMMARY

The "message" on the value of controlling blood sugar in Type 2 diabetes mellitus has been skewed towards drug treatments by both medical research and advertising. Diabetes is an important independent risk factor for cardiovascular disease, but it is not the "whole story". The first line options to combat glucose intolerance in Syndrome X are the same as preferred options to prevent and treat all components of Syndrome X and they rest to a major degree in lifestyle change and nutritional interventions.

The preferred initial approach to problems with glucose intolerance, insulin resistance and maturity onset diabetes involve lifestyle change, dietary modification and the use of selected dietary supplements that may assist in lowering blood sugar (see Sections 7 and 8). New information seems to reinforce the idea that drugs used to treat Type 2 diabetes are best reserved for the individual who does not respond to diet, nutritional interventions and lifestyle change, at least until safe and more effective allopathic interventions emerge.

# SECTION 4:

# COMBAT HYPERTENSION: THE SILENT KILLER

## Risk Factors for Hypertension

The killer constellation of Syndrome X includes the readily identifiable cardiovascular risk factor of high blood pressure. The causes of a sustained rise in blood pressure overlap with the causes of many of the other risk factors of cardiovascular disease. I reiterate that the risk factors within the "bouquet of barbed wire" are highly intertwined. Individuals who are obese, do not exercise, consume excessive salt in their diet and drink alcohol excessively are likely to develop sustained hypertension. Many people with one or more of these characteristics may have Syndrome X. When these lifestyle problems are identified, assessed and aggregated, they involve a consideration of more than 100 million people in the US!

Genetic (hereditary) tendencies seem to play a major role in the causation of hypertension and African or Mexican Americans or individuals with a strong family history of hypertension are at particular risk. Mexican Americans not only have a high incidence of hypertension, but blood pressure treatment is neglected in this group as well. Furthermore, Hispanics, Native American Indians and female African Americans are also at an increased risk for the development of Syndrome X. The evidence that adverse lifestyle promotes sustained hypertension is more obvious when one examines scientific studies which show that weight loss, exercise and reductions in salt or alcohol intake can all prevent the development of high blood pressure. Furthermore, there are other lifestyle changes which may influence the development or presence of hypertension e.g. stress reduction and the elimination of substance abuse, including the abuse of prescription or over-the-counter medicines or dietary supplements.

Conventional medical opinion has tended to question the role of stress or poor nutrition in the causation of hypertension. Some medical literature tends to classify these factors as inconsistent in their effect on high blood pressure or of doubtful benefit when reversed. However, I believe strongly that scientific literature directs us to the importance of stress reduction and nutritional interventions in both the prevention and treatment of high blood pressure. These important interventions include stress management by lifestyle change, appropriate control of the dietary intake of salt, sugar, potassium, calcium, magnesium, soluble dietary fiber (especially beta glucan types of soluble fiber), fish oil and other selected nutritional factors.

## THE SILENT KILLER IS OFTEN MILD

Almost two million adults in North America will develop high blood pressure on an annual basis and the occurrence of hypertension increases with age. Hypertension has been commonly referred to as the "silent killer", but Syndrome X may be more deserving of this onerous label. Not only does Syndrome X act as a silent killer, it is present as a "hidden" epidemic. We have learned that insulin resistance (hyperinsulinism) and high blood pressure are closely related, in a presumed cause and effect manner.

There have been problems in the definition of clinical hypertension because a single or isolated blood pressure recording during screening cannot be taken as evidence of high blood pressure. It is generally accepted that high blood pressure exists if there is a recording of a systolic blood pressure of greater than 140 millimeters of mercury (mmHg) or a diastolic blood pressure of greater than 85 mmHg. However, blood pressure does change in response to various stimuli and surges or increases in blood pressure are normal during physical activity. Modest alterations in blood pressure are normal events in day to day activity. Continuous monitoring of blood pressure during normal day to day activity is an important research tool which may assist in relating metabolic changes in Syndrome X to changes in systemic blood pressure. More research observations of these relationships are awaited.

## MAKING A DIAGNOSIS OF HYPERTENSION

Before hypertension is diagnosed, the elevation of blood pressure should be demonstrated to be sustained. It is well recognized that an individual who may be anxious during clinical examination may have an initial elevation of the blood pressure on a first recording. Therefore, many clinicians have the subject at rest, in a lying position, prior to measurements of blood pressure. To be certain that high blood pressure is present, it is advisable to take blood pressure on more than one occasion.

It is possible for the systolic blood pressure to be elevated alone and this is termed "isolated systolic hypertension". There is a risk to health with isolated systolic hypertension, but it seems to be less than the cardiovascular risks associated with occurrences of both systolic and diastolic elevations of blood pressure. It is clear that elevated blood pressure is more common in African or Mexican Americans, especially in men below the age of 55 years. High blood pressure is noted more often in all men over the age of 55 years, especially in those who belong to lower socioeconomic groups.

Several large organizations have provided statistics on the incidence and prevalence (occurrence) of high blood pressure. It is apparent that of all subjects with high blood pressure, at least three-quarters have "mild hypertension" (stage 1 hypertension). Hypertension is generally accepted to be blood pressure readings with a systolic measurement of greater than 140 to 159 mmHg together diastolic blood pressure readings of greater than 90 to 99 mmHg. The vast majority of treatment decisions that are made by healthcare givers involve the treatment of mild hypertension. In simple terms, the chances are that an individual with newly-diagnosed high blood pressure will often have mild disease. Many people with Syndrome X have mild hypertension. It is important to note that mild disease may often be missed and it is most amenable to correction by natural measures or lifestyle changes, not by the rapid stroke of the prescription pen.

## THE HIGHER THE BLOOD PRESSURE THE GREATER THE RISK

The advantages of reducing mild elevations of blood pressure are not quite as obvious as the advantages that result from the reduction of moderate or severe hypertension. By taking information from many different clinical trials of blood pressure lowering, it has been demonstrated that there is an overall reduction of 10% or more in death rate from coronary artery disease by the effective treatment of moderate hypertension.

## HOW IS INSULIN RESISTANCE (SYNDROME X) RELATED TO HYPERTENSION?

There are now many studies in the scientific literature which show that insulin resistance and high blood levels of insulin are associated with elevations of blood pressure. Studies of families indicate that close relatives of people with hypertension tend to exhibit insulin resistance compared with those who do not have a family history of high blood pressure. Important studies, performed more than ten years ago, defined the association of high blood insulin levels and high blood pressure (Hypertension, 20, 797, 1992).

Observations on the development of hypertension imply that individuals with high blood insulin levels are more likely to develop high blood pressure over a period of time. It is suspected that two thirds of all people with high blood pressure may have one or more other components of Syndrome X, especially resistance to the actions of insulin with a corresponding increase in blood insulin levels (compensatory hyperinsulinemia). The components of Syndrome X gang together to increase risks of heart attack, stroke and vascular disease, including poor circulation to the extremities of the body. There is no doubt that people with "full blown" Syndrome X who have established hypertension have the greatest risks of cardiovascular disease.

The precise reason why insulin resistance with compensatory increases in blood insulin levels cause high blood pressure are not fully understood. It is known that insulin works to amplify the effects of certain body hormones (secreted by the adrenal glands) that cause blood vessels to contract (constrict). These are the "stress" hormones (epinephrine and other catecholamines). One likely explanation of the relationship is the effect of insulin on the amount of salt (sodium chloride) that exists in the body. Insulin can work to make the kidneys retain excessive salt in the body. Later in this section of the book, I discuss the role of salt intake as a cause of hypertension. An important characteristic of people with Syndrome X is the sensitivity they develop to extra salt in their diet. More salt in the diet causes more salt retention by the body which results in an increase in body water and a rise in blood pressure. The importance of salt restriction in the combat against Syndrome X diet is very important and often underemphasized.

## OVERDOING DRUG TREATMENTS FOR HYPERTENSION?

Overall, there may have been tendency to use drug therapy to treat mild hypertension at the expense of considering more "natural" options to control blood pressure (déjà vu). This line of reasoning concerning drug treatments is purposefully monotonous in this book. It is recognized that about 60 - 70 million Americans may have hypertension of variable severity. As a consequence, many healthcare agencies and government institutions have promoted programs for screening for high blood pressure and political initiatives have proposed public health projects such as the National High Blood Pressure Education Program. This widespread level of interest in reducing blood pressure has resulted in improvements in the management of hypertension, but it may have also resulted in the widespread "premature" use of drug therapy to lower blood pressure.

Lifestyle changes or other natural methods of blood pressure reduction may be regarded as safe and effective, in a cost-beneficial manner, but they do not usually figure strongly in standard medical practice. Lowering blood pressure with drugs in the absence of exercising the first line options of lifestyle change has been regarded as "poor medicine". The same reasoning applies to other cardinal components of Syndrome X, notably high blood cholesterol, obesity and insulin resistance (diabetes mellitus).

## GOOD TRENDS HIDE BAD SITUATIONS

The prevalence of high blood pressure in adults seems to have been reduced in the past ten years. This can be attributed largely to public awareness and the increasing application of appropriate lifestyle modification to lower blood pressure. This reduction in blood pressure cannot be solely attributed to any specific medical advances and it is certainly not a complete or totally direct consequence of the prescription of blood pressure lowering medications.

Surveys have shown that there is an increasing level of awareness about the consequences of high blood pressure and people are becoming better educated in methods to lower blood pressure. The level of awareness of the negative health consequences of high blood pressure has been estimated over the past twenty years to have improved from a level of about 50% to a level of about 80%. Whilst the awareness of elevated blood pressure in adults and its negative consequences have increased, the alarming increase in blood pressure in children and adolescents has not received great attention. Hypertensive children become hypertensive adults and many of these individuals are incubating Syndrome X. Coincidental with an increasing level of awareness and increasing control of blood pressure in adults is an enormous increase in the number of individuals receiving drug treatment for blood pressure. People with hypertension receiving drug therapy for high blood pressure have increased over the past 20 years from about 35% to about 75%. This situation is both good and bad!

I am not rejecting the opinion that many of these people with high blood pressure require drug treatment, but I question whether or not there exists among these people a significant group of individuals who are receiving drug therapy for hypertension who could have managed their disease by more natural options or positive lifestyle changes. The application of "natural options" could potentially obviate the need for the prescription of blood pressure lowering medicines in some individuals; or at least reduce the dosage requirements of these medications. Since the adverse effects of many antihypertensive drugs are often dosage related, this is a clear advantage.

## Benefits of Lowering Blood Pressure

Improvements in blood pressure control have been linked incompletely to the findings that there has been a 50% decline in death rate from strokes and about a 40% reduction in deaths from coronary artery disease over the past 20 years. These statistics sound reassuring, but it should be recognized that cardiovascular deaths, taken in composite, are still so common that they account for a number of deaths that remains almost equal to the sum total of deaths from all other causes. Thus, over-optimistic assessments of these trends could be used to conceal a situation for which there is great residual concern. Whatever the advances in the management of hypertension have been over the past two decades, there still remains a lot of ground to cover in controlling (preventing and treating) the important cardiovascular risk factor of high blood pressure. It is important to realize that dealing with insulin resistance (Syndrome X) has not been identified as synonymous with controlling hypertension. This may be a partial medical mistake !

There is no question that elevated arterial blood pressure is a principle risk factor for both coronary artery disease and cerebrovascular accident (stroke). In early studies of controlling blood pressure, there was some difficulty in demonstrating that lowering blood pressure had any real benefit in reducing the occurrence of coronary artery disease. However, these "preventive" clinical trials did show clear benefits in the reduction of stroke and renal disease. More recent studies have indicated that reductions in blood pressure reduce the occurrence of coronary artery disease, especially in elderly individuals. Again, the difficulty in showing the benefit of impacting one component of Syndrome X (or "the bouquet of barbed wire") underscores the concept of attacking all of the disorders within Syndrome X (déjà vu).

## Side Effects of Anti-hypertensive Drugs

The principle reason for a failure of some of the earlier preventive anti-hypertensive drug trials to show benefits in the reduction of coronary artery disease may have been due lack of compliance with medication or due (directly or indirectly) to some of the adverse effects of the blood pressure lowering medications used in the clinical trials. It may be surprizing to some readers that blood pressure lowering drugs can be linked on occasion to cardiovascular disabilities and death. The use of "water pills" (thiazide diuretics) has been examined in this respect. Thiazide diuretics may have a number of adverse effects including alterations of body chemicals with a resulting low serum potassium and magnesium. In addition, these diuretics (water pills) may contribute to abnormalities of blood lipids and glucose metabolism. Thus, these drugs can sometimes make Syndrome X worse, and by inference they may enhance cardiovascular risk in some circumstances.

On occasion, thiazide diuretics have been associated with the precipitation of diabetes mellitus and even cardiac arrhythmias. There is continuing argument about the safety of some antihypertensive drugs (blood pressure-lowering medication) and this has resulted in a tendency for physicians to use blood pressure-lowering medication with "safer profiles". However, blood pressure lowering medication is often limited in its use by side effects in general, and these factors have encouraged the exploration of more natural or safer approaches to blood pressure reduction.

To discuss all the adverse effects of blood pressure lowering medication is not possible because of the vast number of actual or potential side effects of these medications. Indeed, a detailed discussion of every side effect of every blood pressure lowering drug may serve as a disincentive to anyone taking antihypertensive medication. It is certainly not my intent to advise anyone to stop drug therapy for high blood pressure, but therapy must occur on an "all facts known basis". Anti-hypertensive drugs tend to be expensive and evidence exists that more than one-third of all people taking blood pressure medication experience difficulty in paying for the medication. The situation can be overcome to some degree by selecting generic drugs, providing such drugs are known to have equivalence in their therapeutic effect to "standard" brands of drugs (similar actions and benefits). Using a generic drug rather than a branded drug, sometimes reduces the cost of therapy of hypertension by 75%. Anyone who is taking multiple drug therapy needs to educate themselves more about the value of "combination therapy", especially if the combination approach can incorporate complementary, natural options.

## THE COMPLIANCE PROBLEM

It is alarming to note that up to one in five people receiving anti-hypertensive therapy may cease taking medication because of side effects. One important issue is that lowering blood pressure should not significantly interfere with quality of life and, fortunately, newer drugs have been developed with more acceptable side effect profiles. Despite this, some people with high blood pressure are still using obsolete and in some circumstances dangerous anti-hypertensive medications. Several classes of drugs are popular for lowering blood pressure. These drugs include: mild acting diuretics, a class of compounds called angiotensin converting enzyme inhibitors, known commonly as ACE inhibitors, drugs that block calcium channels and "beta-blocking" drugs. However, "beta-blocker" drugs may tend to block the actions of insulin and their use in states of insulin resistance and Syndrome X requires continuing reappraisal. Anti-hypertensive drugs that tend to result in orthostatic hypotension (profound fall in blood pressure when changing posture) are best avoided, especially in the elderly.

Aside from the unpleasant physical effects of poorly controlled lowering of blood pressure to subnormal levels (postural hypotension), anti-hypertensive drugs are very common causes of mood disturbance, impairment of sexual activity, and a decrease in psychomotor (brain) function. It is very problematic when blood pressure lowering drugs interfere with an individual's ability to undertake an exercise program. When a physician tries to treat an asymptomatic disease like hypertension (the "silent killer") with drugs that cause unpleasant symptoms, there will always be a tendency for people to consider the therapy to be worse than the disease (compare with lowering blood cholesterol with drugs, discussed in Section 2). This is a major challenge for the healthcare giver. However, it is a further reason for the healthcare giver and the hypertensive individual to try and adopt more acceptable, gentler and more natural solutions to the therapy of high blood pressure; without jumping prematurely to drug treatment and its frequent association with onerous side effects.

I accept that "natural options" which include lifestyle change, diet and the use of nutraceuticals may not always achieve the desired outcome, but they can be "adjunctive" to allopathic treatments in many cases. If a natural option can only reduce the dosage requirements of some antihypertensive drugs, then they are a real contribution to care. It is recognized that the side effects of many drugs are dose dependent and options that reduce drug dosages can be very valuable complementary therapies (déjà vu).

## Causes of Stubbornly High Blood Pressure

An important consideration in the assessment of the effectiveness of any program for the treatment of high blood pressure is the recognition that there are many circumstances that can interfere with methods to lower blood pressure. An individual with high blood pressure is not advised to self-medicate and he or she should be aware of interactions between drugs (and foods and dietary supplements) that lower blood pressure. There are many over-the-counter medications or dietary supplements that should be avoided in the person with elevated blood pressure; because these agents may promote high blood pressure or they can interfere with anti-hypertensive drugs. Table 19 gives a list of circumstances that may interfere with blood pressure lowering interventions.

- Lack of compliance with treatment
- Weight gain
- Salt excess in diet
- Excessive stress
- Substance abuse (or its withdrawal)
- Medication that increases blood pressure, e.g. non-steroidal anti-inflammatory drugs, steroids, hormonal replacement therapy, salt containing anti-acids, decongestant remedies slimming drugs and other commonly used drugs.
- Use of some dangerous dietary supplements, e.g., those containing ephedra or botanicals that are known to cause significant raises in blood pressure.

**Table 19:** Circumstances that may interfere with natural options or drug therapy to control blood pressure. Note: some of the problems occur as a result of the injudicious use of "natural options".

## LOWERING OF BLOOD PRESSURE WITHOUT DRUGS

Many individuals have taken anti-hypertensive medication prematurely without the application of non-pharmacologic (non-drug) approaches. Why? Physicians and patients are encouraged appropriately to apply treatment methods for which there is very hard and fast evidence of a benefit as shown by their performance in controlled clinical trials. Table 20 summarizes some of the more important non-drug options available to reduce blood pressure, but they may not have been backed by the kind of rigorous research which is performed to show "drug effectiveness". In some cases their effectiveness is questionable.

Most non-drug options for controlling high blood pressure include significant changes in lifestyle which are common to the interventions that will decrease the risks of cardiovascular disease. In other words, they combat Syndrome X. It has been suggested that "non-pharmacologic" therapies are difficult for a medical practitioner to include in the treatment of mild hypertension because of compliance problems. However, part of the therapy of mild hypertension should be an attempt to motivate a patient to engage in lifestyle change and encourage the belief that it is possible to use multiple natural options together as a first-line management strategy for mild hypertension.

**Some Natural Blood Pressure Lowering Agents or Options**

- Decreased sodium intake
- Optimal potassium intake
- Optimal zinc intake
- Niacin
- Vitamin C
- Essential fatty acids
- Bioflavonoids
- Mushrooms (shiitake)
- Taurine
- Co-emzyme Q10
- Mistletoe (Viscum album)
- Black Cohosh (Cimicifuga racemosa)
- Hawthorne

- Calcium
- Magnesium
- Celery
- Berry extracts

**Table 20**: Nutrients and natural agents that have been described as capable of lowering elevated blood pressure. Individuals with high blood pressure are recommended to seek medical advice and attention. Individuals with hypertension should not self-medicate to lower their own blood pressure. Not all listed options are known to be safe and effective.

## EXERCISE AND BLOOD PRESSURE

Scrutiny of a very important study performed by the Joint National Committee on Detection, Evaluation and Treatment of High Blood Pressure (JNC) should motivate people to re-examine the links between lifestyle and high blood pressure. In 1993, an important report was made in the medical journal, Archives of Internal Medicine (The Fifth Report of the Joint National Committee on Detection, Evaluation and Treatment of High Blood Pressure). This document recommended that all patients with high blood pressure be recommended to engage in regular physical exercise.

Evidence has been produced that exercise may in itself control hypertension and it has the added advantage of permitting a reduction in the amount of drug therapy that may be required to control blood pressure. It is apparent that all types of physical exercise may be beneficial, including simple activity, such as cleaning or household chores. Of course, optimum cardiovascular conditioning occurs usually as a result of more strenuous types of exercise which should be undertaken with the supervision of healthcare givers or professional trainers. In mature individuals, an exercise program must be preceded by an assessment of the risks of exercise and it is best applied with care.

## ELIMINATING STRESS

Stress reduction techniques have been shown in well controlled clinical trials to have beneficial effects on the reduction of cardiovascular risk factors, but their use as a primary method for controlling blood pressure has remained somewhat in question. A lack of consistent demonstration of stress reduction or behavioral techniques to reduce blood pressure should not prevent a healthcare giver from recommending this type of intervention because stress reduction has multiple health benefits. There is much to be gained from stress reduction in terms of improving a patient's well-being and decreasing cardiovascular risk overall. "Alternative" medicine is an ideal way of reducing stress by the applications of treatment disciplines such as biofeedback, hypnosis, coping skills and Yoga.

## DIETARY SUPPLEMENTS EMERGE AS AN OPTION

The role of nutritional interventions to lower blood pressure continues to be questioned by many medical practitioners. Unfortunately, some people with this disbelief of the benefit of a nutritional approach do not take the trouble to examine the evidence for a benefit, even though the available evidence may be "small" in comparison to drug research. The use of remedies of natural origin (especially herbs) to lower blood pressure should be applied with medical supervision (Table 20).

Dietary supplements such as fish oil preparations, garlic and mineral supplements are known to lower blood pressure in a variety of circumstances. It is argued that the gastrointestinal side effects of fish oil intake in the diet may counteract the overall benefit of this intervention. However, in the commonplace situation of omega-3 fatty acid deficiency, this argument is not tenable given the availability of deodorized, concentrated or enteric coated fish oil capsules (OligOmega™, CardiOmega, DiabOmega™, OmEPA™ greater than 70% EPA concentrate of fish oil). Arguments that low caffeine diets cannot be clearly shown to control hypertension are not to be used as reasons to ignore excessive caffeine inclusion in the diet. Caffeine is known in many daily settings to cause elevations in blood pressure. It is suggested that elevations of blood pressure due to caffeine are short-lived or quite transient, but the dietary intake of caffeine is frequently continuous in many people. We are a nation with many habitual cola or coffee drinkers. "Pepsi, Coke, Soda Pop and Cola" are a challenge to cardiovascular health (sugar and caffeine.)

## Salt and Blood Pressure

Up to one-half of all people may be able to raise their blood pressure significantly by exceeding normal daily intakes of salt (sodium chloride). The role of excessive salt intake in blood pressure control is well known and anyone with high blood pressure is advised to avoid excessive salt intake. The addition of salt (sodium chloride) to food is a learned habit which can be broken with effort. It has been described as a habit "most people can't shake". Recently, limited evidence has emerged that taking salt in the diet from more natural sources may have some benefits. However, the body recognizes salt as salt and I find it difficult to believe that natural sources of salt have a great deal to offer in protecting the body from the blood pressure elevating effects of salt, per se.

The best way to break the salt habit may not be just to quit using salt but to replace it in culinary activities with well selected, tasty herbs and spices. A number of true "salt substitute" products are available that contain no salt. However, one should be aware that a number of "salt substitutes" contain salt (sodium chloride). The most creative combinations of spices and herbs that can be used as salt substitutes include: onions, garlic, peppers, citrus peel, carrots, oregano, celery seed, marjoram, thyme, cumin, coriander, mustard and rosemary. The adventurous salt-substituter has the option of mixing their own spice concoction to assist in "kicking" the salt habit. Salt intake must be controlled in the combat against Syndrome X, given the enhanced sensitivity to salt that exists in this disorder.

## Summarizing Natural Approaches to Blood Pressure Reduction

My proposal that that narrowly focused interventions are not worthy objectives in decreasing cardiovascular risk applies in the management of hypertension. Just lowering blood pressure may be equally as misguided as just lowering cholesterol. Interventions to reduce cardiovascular risks should occur together and these risks often go hand-in-hand. The importance of combating the components of Syndrome X together emerges again and again. I stress that I am not rejecting conventional medical approaches to the treatment of hypertension, where such treatment is appropriately indicated, but I am pointing out that a number people may opt for a drug treatment approach at the expense of considering other effective, but more gentle options. Table 21 summarizes some approaches to hypertension, applying conventional approaches and remedies of natural origin. These approaches are best used under supervision and it should be noted that remedies of natural origin can interact with blood pressure lowering drugs and each other.

- Weight reduction
- Restriction of sodium in the diet
- Physical exercise
- Stress reduction
- Dietary modification and use of dietary supplements e.g., calcium, fish oil, magnesium potassium, beta glucans from oats, soy protein and garlic
- Specific pharmaceutical options
- Addressing insulin resistance (Syndrome X)

**Table 21:** Lifestyle or natural options available to reduce blood pressure that, in the author's options, should be considered among first line therapy for high blood pressure. Specific pharmaceutical options are important, but they may not always be the first line approach.

## CHAPTER SUMMARY

Self-medication is not recommended in the management of significant degrees of hypertension. Of all known factors in the cause of high blood pressure, the correction of insulin resistance (the pivotal component of Syndrome X) requires greater attention in medical practice. Whilst it has not been conclusively demonstrated that controlling insulin resistance lowers blood pressure consistently, weight control is often effective. Table 22 summarizes an approach to the management of hypertension that is more "lifestyle-based" than some conventional medical strategies. Blood pressure lowering medication is an important area of continuing innovation that has saved lives and improved well-being; but it is best used after exhausting simple and gentle options to lower blood pressure in cases of mild hypertension and it can improve blood pressure control in moderate and severe hypertension, where drug treatment is mandatory. (Table 22)

## LIFESTYLE MODIFICATIONS:

- Control weight
- Elimination of substance abuse
- Exercise
- Dietary change
- Supplements e.g. beta glucan, oat soluble fiber extracts, soy protein with fermented components, fish oil, good mineral balance etc.
- Smoking cessation
- Address insulin resistance where present ("Think" Syndrome X).

## LIFESTYLE CHANGE

| | |
|---|---|
| Good response | Good response requires a followup program to reinforce the change in behaviors |
| No response | Assess whether or not there has been a change in lifestyle and compliance with advice. Go do drugs? |
| No compliance | Repeat lifestyle advice and intervention Go do drugs? |

**Table 22:** This table summarizes a treatment approach to mild hypertension but its recommendation are relevant to moderate and severe hypertension. Note that it is expanded to incorporate strategies to combat Syndrome X and other cardiovascular risk factors. Most cases of newly diagnosed hypertension are mild and the emphasis is placed upon natural options. Drug therapy of increasing intensity and variety is best reserved, where possible, for moderate or severe forms of hypertension that are recalcitrant to simple interventions.

# SECTION 5

# OBESITY AND
# THE SLIM CHANCE

## DISPELLING THE FANTASIES

Many people can shed a few pounds in the short term, but few obese individuals maintain their weight loss targets. This book is not a series of pretty pictures, nor does it contain a series of false promises. Fad diets and weight loss tricks emerge with regularity, as do new cases of significant obesity. I cannot apologize for asking people to face the reality that weight control remains an unresolved but highly significant public health initiative in all Western nations. It may distress some readers to know that "all calories count" or "eat what you like and grow thin" is an absurd contention. Moving into some "Zone" of metabolic fantasy has not been universally effective and liberal intake of fat for weight loss is not a healthy "Diet Revolution", even though some aspects of these approaches may be a move in the right direction.

Losing weight involves calorie control for most people, but lifestyle change and behavior modification are just as important, if successful weight control is to be achieved. Many Americans are strangers to healthy lifestyle, and few people question their own abundant, dietary excesses. Perhaps the most important point to make is that there is no single diet or dietary approach that is universal in its potential benefits for health or weight control (déjà vu). There is great metabolic variation among individuals and dietary intakes require certain tailoring to special needs. In logical terms, why would one be naïve enough to believe that there is one lifestyle or one diet that will work for a problem in society, such as obesity, that has so many complex causes.

Some nutrition researchers have talked about the "no diet option", but they have to focus still on the importance of calorie intake, exercise and behavior modification. Losing weight while you read this book, or while you sleep as a consequence of reading this book, will not occur. It is time to go back to basics, forget the nonsense and throw away the current dietary fads and fallacies that have served little purpose other than to cause massive confusion. In the words of an anonymous mentor, "Pigs can fly but they are rare birds !"

## NOT ANOTHER DIET!

As we enter the new millennium, we leave a century behind of multiple dietary renaissances which have led to a growing interest in "food as medicine". The 20th century bred many confusing recommendations for "new diets", but few if any of the diets were "new" and none could be perceived as "holistic" for health. The large number of "different diets" that have been recommended is sure testimony to the fact that not one alone has presented a pathway to global health or even sustained weight loss.

The reason for this situation is quite simple. People are different with different nutritional needs at different times in their lives, under different circumstances. Thus, diets have to be tailored to an individuals' needs and when diets are used in isolation of overall changes in lifestyle they can be quite useless, or even harmful. Again, one needs to broaden the horizon on health maintenance, beyond the simple concept of a fixed dietary regimen.

## RHETORIC ON DIETS

The concept of the "ideal diet" is constantly in question and a focus on the "no-diet" option has to incorporate the notion of "healthy eating". Everyone talks about optimal nutrition which defies a consensus definition and few individuals can comply with the "ideal diet" (if it exists). This dilemma may be amenable to a limited solution by the use of well chosen dietary guidelines with or without the addition of some dietary supplements, but this approach is not a practical long term strategy. Whilst one could be criticized for the approach of supplementing an existing diet, rather than attempting a healthy modification of the diet, it is obvious that even the most dedicated homemaker would have difficulty in finding, preparing and affording an "optimal" diet for a family. This conundrum gets worse as the "food industry" purveys more and more types of "attractive" but unhealthy, "processed" foods. A nutritional program to combat Syndrome X and cardiovascular disease, whilst promoting health in general, rests in a consideration of basic dietary principles and it involves the dissolution of dietary "myths and fallacies".

A healthy diet must address general health by definition, not merely one issue in isolation. For example, looking at a diet that is designed just to lower cholesterol is problematic, but hospital manuals of specific diets for "this and that" are often rigidly applied. The human body can manufacture at least one and one-half grams of cholesterol per day. If diets low in cholesterol are selected, then the body will compensate in many subjects (about 50% of all individuals) by increasing the endogenous (inside the body) synthesis of cholesterol. This factor makes a low cholesterol diet alone a less effective means of reducing total blood cholesterol than many people may have presupposed. The significance of this example of the limitations of a diet focused on lowering cholesterol alone can be applied to the shortcomings of a diet for obesity management alone, for skin health alone etc.

## What Causes Obesity?

Predictably, the answer to this question is very far from simple. However, the consumer of weight loss plans, books or products must have insight into the science of obesity in order to make an informed choice of a weight control program. Understanding why one may be fat is a major step in the battle to get thinner. This educational approach is omitted from many popular weight loss books or "novels" and pages of menus in weight loss books are rarely followed, and sometimes they are not the thoughts or work of the author of the book. If we accept the need to tailor diets to individual needs, then menu plans must be questioned. Using nutri-

tional principles obtained by self-education is the best way to have
a person engage in a weight control program

Obesity occurs when the net amount of energy intake into the
body is greater than the net utilization of energy by the body over a
period of time. Some practitioners of alternative medicine "choke"
on these established principles. Obesity is age dependent and the
peak prevalence (occurrence) of obesity occurs in Western countries
usually between the age of 55 and 65, when at least one half of all
women and one third of all men are overweight. The risk factors
for obesity in females and males of these age groups have been
defined to some degree. A female is more likely to be fat during her
mature years if she has had more than three pregnancies, is not mar-
ried and is of lower socioeconomic status. Both genetic and environmental factors play a variable role in the causation of obesity.

Genetic or familial differences determine how people handle energy intake and the utilization of energy by the body is an
important consideration. Overall, the most common and important
determinant of obesity is "overeating". This overeating is controlled or not controlled by complex behavioral factors. These
facts mean that dieting cannot be successful in the intermediate to
long-term without behavioral changes that influence eating habits.

There are some special circumstances in which obesity
occurs. The climacteric (menopausal period) often heralds the onset
of weight gain for females. In addition, the less well defined or recognized "male menopause" (andropause) often signals weight gain
in the male. These circumstances of weight gain can be approached
in an effective manner but require sustained dietary intervention
with special care to provide nutritional principles that both address
weight control and help prevent chronic degenerative diseases in the
mature adult. Carefully performed studies of body composition
show that the amount of fat compared with the amount of muscle
present in the body changes with age, with a move towards the
body having more fat with advancing years.

Obesity in childhood is notoriously difficult to treat and
many standard dietary interventions to control weight almost
always fail. The outcome of the treatment of established obesity in
children is so miserable that weight stabilization is often the medical target. Thus, prevention of excessive weight gain in children is
a key, unfulfilled public health concern. Obese children are disad-

vantaged and often emotionally upset. These children are at significant risk of social and medical problems and obese children often become obese adults. Most "successful" dietary interventions in children result only in prevention of further weight gain, rather than weight loss. I reiterate that there is an alarming increase in diabetes mellitus in children and this diabetes is emerging as the type that most often occurs in the mature adult (type 2 diabetes or maturity onset diabetes of the young, MODY), where obesity plays a major role.

## A Reasonable Composite Diet

There are increasing numbers of popular books on weight loss which provide menus or recipes that serve little purpose and some published menus do not even match the authors' recommendations. The successful controller of weight is the individual that can take the basic principles of nutrition for weight control and apply them in their day to day activity. Some people will say "I followed the plan but it did not work". Often, these people do not understand the basis of the plan and everyday life does not permit their attempts to eat by fixed menus. Furthermore, without lifestyle adjustments including modification of behavior and engagement in exercise to burn calories weight control cannot be sustained. On this basis, I urge readers to grasp the basics of nutrition, because the combat against obesity is these days "back to basics".

Individuals can think in food groups which are composed traditionally of four categories, including: the meat or vegetable protein group, the dairy group, the fruit and vegetable group, and the grain group. It is generally accepted that most adults need a couple of servings from the meat-protein and dairy groups together with at least four (or five) servings from the vegetable-fruit and grain groups. It sounds simple but the average American diet bears no resemblance to these basic recommendations, even accepting that these recommendations may not be "ideal". The USDA pyramid recommends certain eating patterns, but its recommendations have been hammered by criticisms in recent times. The "pyramid" is too slanted towards the inclusion of refined carbohydrates and it is deficient in clear recommendations for healthy types of fat. I believe that the recommendations of the Food Pyramid combined with an election of some people to become vegetarian has created a number of "obese vegetarians" with Syndrome X.

Our habits concerning the consumption of meat-protein is worthy of analysis. Red meat is often high in saturated fat and cholesterol. It is best used in moderation until blood lipids (fats) are controlled, when infrequent inclusions of lean red meat or "white meat" in the diet may be "harmless". Poultry and fish are preferred to red meat for dietary inclusion in the healthy cardiovascular diet. It is often stated that fat should always be trimmed from sources of protein. Whilst this is true for poultry and meat, the fat on fish is abundant in health-giving omega 3, essential fatty acids (good fats). There is a danger in stating that poultry is healthier food than red meat or pork. When it comes to weight control and cardiovascular health a piece of fried chicken bearing its skin is just as bad as the greasiest pork or beef chop.

The desirable forms of protein in our diet have been redefined with much more emphasis being placed on the incorporation of vegetable protein into the diet. Vegetable protein is often equally as nutritious as animal protein and it makes more ecological sense. For example, feeding tons of soy protein to cows to produce a few pounds of meat protein just does not make sense, especially when one considers that soy protein is good for health. Moving towards vegetable protein inclusion in the diet, especially of soy origin, at the expense of animal protein has been associated with a plethora of health benefits. These benefits are discussed in detail in my book entitled "The Soy Revolution", Dell Publishing, NY, 2000. Soy food, when taken in the correct format has a low glycemic index, is devoid of saturated fat and careful research studies show that soy protein can actually lower "bad types" blood cholesterol (notably LDL and triglycerides).

Whole dairy products are best limited in a diet that is planned to promote cardiovascular wellness because they present a cholesterol and saturated fat burden. Milk is an excellent source of protein, fat soluble vitamins (A and D) and calcium. These important, nutritious components of milk are available in low fat dairy products which are to be preferred by the individual who seeks cardiovascular health. The food industry is now focused on making "healthy milk" by reducing its undesirable components and adding "nutraceuticals" such as soluble fiber or beta glucans from soluble oat fiber. This is an example of "functional beverages" (Bravo Foods Inc., Palm Beach, Florida).

There has been a tendency to both overestimate and underestimate the nutritional value of dairy products. This has led to massive consumer confusion with parents wondering whether or not they should hold back on milk intake in their children. The menopausal female who is looking for extra calcium and vitamin D to ward off osteoporosis may inadvertently avoid milk because of thoughts of excessive calorie intake and excessive saturated fat intake that have been associated with weight gain. These issues are discussed later in this book as questions that are answered: "Is Milk Healthy?" and "Making Milk Healthy".

The fruit-vegetable and grain groups are highly desirable components of a diet for cardiovascular health. The only limitation to this aspect of the diet is to watch total calorie intake. An individual with a "big appetite" (high satiety level) is advised to fill up with vegetables that have a low calorie density (and a low glycemic index). The concept of caloric density of food is important. Certain foods are more "dilute" in calories than others because of their variable makeup of protein, fat, carbohydrate and fiber. Fiber-rich foods are generally "dilute" in calories and will help promote satiety (a feeling of fullness in the stomach). Fiber is the archetypal food with a low glycemic index and this makes fiber rich foods very valuable in the fight against Syndrome X (see Section 8 on beta glucans and the secret of soluble fiber). Excessive calories from simple sugars or refined carbohydrates are readily converted into saturated fat in the body and they gyrate blood sugar. Simple sugars are the key enemy in the fight against Syndrome X.

One hallmark of the unhealthy American diet is the over-inclusion of refined carbohydrates which is tantamount, in "metabolic weight control terms", to eating excess saturated fat. I reiterate that simple sugars in the diet are readily converted to body fat. We have learned that the tendency to exclude dietary fat and promote carbohydrate intake is a popular, but ineffective, method of weight loss that has been proposed erroneously by the uninformed as a good pathway to weight loss. This is the basis of the "low fat con" promoted by the food industry who forgot to mention that low fat does not mean low calories. Indeed, the "low fat" claim may often mean high simple sugar intake. If carbohydrates are included to a major degree in any diet, they should be preferentially derived from complex carbohydrates which are found in foods that contain more dietary fiber, vitamins, minerals and essential fats (omega 3 and 6 fatty acids). Complex carbohydrates and fiber are most ubiquitous in "fibrous" vegetables and fruits. If the fruit and vegetables one eats do not require "a good chew", then they may not be healthful.

A special and repetitive mention of grains and cereals is necessary. Overall, these foods are an excellent source of dietary fiber with all of its known health giving benefits and fiber is non-calorigenic with an ability to promote satiety (a feeling of fullness that is useful for those people who are controlling calories in their diet). The recognition of the benefits of dietary fiber for health have resulted in increasing consumption of breakfast cereals. Unfortunately, many popular breakfast cereals are laced with sugar in a manner that overrides any beneficial effect of their fiber content. In addition, the modern "breakfast pastry" or "pop-tart" is a sinister ally of Syndrome X. Americans number one cause of "roller coaster" blood sugar may be the sugar-laced cereal or breakfast pastry with the morning coffee.

## Main Dietary Constituents in Simple Forms

Glucose is an immediately available source of energy for cells. Although glucose can be stored as glycogen in the liver and muscle tissue, this store is quite small and provides only approximately 2,500 calories of immediate energy. This energy store is rapidly utilized during strenuous exercise. In contrast, fats have a higher energy potential and produce two times as many calories on a weight per weight basis compared with carbohydrates or proteins. Thus, fat stores within the body are the greatest source of energy. The body of a male of optimal weight is about 16% fat with a potential energy yield of more than 100,000 calories. We have learned that as we grow older relatively more of our body is composed of fat and most women have more fat than men. Age tends to be associated with inactivity in many people and the breach of the "energy in and energy out", calorie equation piles on the "beef" (fat).

Proteins are a source of nitrogen and they are composed of amino acids. For many years it was believed that eggs and meat were the most ideal source of protein. Fifty years ago the United Nations Committee on Food and Agriculture indicated that eggs provided the best balance of essential amino acids and this outdated message still prevails. These concepts have been superseded as the importance of the constituents (amino acid profile) of proteins for health have become increasingly understood. Evidence exists that vegetable protein, such as soy protein, is quite complete from a nutritional stance and it may be more healthful than animal protein. These matters are discussed in detail in my book "The Soy Revolution".

## UNDERSTANDING VITAMINS

Overall, vitamins are essential for body functions and they facilitate many chemical reactions in the body. Vitamins are generally classified into two groups which include the fat soluble vitamins A, D, E and K and the water soluble vitamins which comprise the vitamin B complex and vitamin C. I shall present a short overview of the main components of food to permit those individuals without a basic knowledge of physiology or nutrition to further understand valuable nutritional interventions for Syndrome X and the promotion of cardiovascular wellness. I stress that this minor overview of nutrition is designed to help the person interested in weight control to engage in healthy a weight control plan in an effective manner, without reaching for a fixed menu plan.

Vitamin A in present in an intact form in fish and meat, or it can be taken indirectly as specific carotenes (carotenoids) in vegetables and fruit. Beta carotene is converted in the body to vitamin A, but this conversion may be impaired in disease states e.g. diabetes mellitus and Syndrome X. Vitamin A is generally important for the structure and function of "epithelial" cells which are located in the skin, the respiratory system, the endocrine system and many parts of the central nervous system. Vitamin A deficiency is practically unknown in Western society and in some respects vitamin A is one of the least important vitamins to supplement in individuals given standard Western diets. However, vitamin A is quite toxic in large doses and it should be used with caution in individuals with liver disease. Vitamin D is characterized by the occurrence of several subtypes, including vitamin D2 (ergosterol), calciferol and vitamin

D3. Vitamin D is ubiquitous in fish and meat. Deficiency in vitamin D results in bone disease and too much vitamin D should be
avoided. Supplements containing vitamin D3 at recommended daily
intakes (RDI) are valuable for many mature adults.

Vitamin E (tocopherol) exists in several chemical forms and
is the classic antioxidant vitamin. Vitamin E is found naturally in
many seed oils and it is beneficial for cardiovascular health.
Vitamin K is present in a variety of food and it exerts an important
effect upon the maintenance of normal blood clotting and the
integrity of blood vessels. Supplements containing vitamin K must
be used with care. Of the fat soluble vitamins, vitamin E has
received particular attention in terms of its potential health giving
benefits in coronary heart disease, where it exerts its principle function as an antioxidant. In general, substantial supplementation
with the fat soluble vitamins A, D and especially K, is often reserved
for those individuals who have a poor diet, are on a restrictive
"diet" or have special needs.

In contrast to the fat soluble vitamins which are stored in the
body, vitamins of the B complex and vitamin C are not stored in
the body and require daily intake. For these reasons, daily vitamin
supplements containing vitamin C and B complex vitamins are often
advised by "nutritionally-orientated" physicians. Thiamin is present in a variety of grains, including wheat and it plays an essential
role in the metabolism of carbohydrates. Thiamin acts as a co-
enzyme for the well known pyruvic acid cycle which is involved in
energy production. Riboflavine is also found in grains and its has
effects similar to those of thiamin, but it also seems to be important in the promotion of normal function of epithelial tissue. Niacin
is known to be important in carbohydrate metabolism and it facil-
itates the functioning of thiamin and riboflavine. Niacin can cause
unpleasant reactions when taken in large doses and this vitamin has
been shown to be useful in some studies as a cholesterol-lowering
agent. However, the adverse effects from this vitamin, when used
in substantial doses, often limits its use as a cholesterol-lowering
agent. Biotin which is classified in the B complex appears to have
special benefits in Syndrome X and it appears to enhance the beneficial actions of the micronutrient metal, chromium, on blood glucose and lipid control.

Vitamin C is well recognized as an important vitamin to

supplement in the average diet. Vitamin C is ubiquitous in fresh fruit and green vegetables and its effects include facilitation of the absorption of iron, actions in the transport of oxygen within the body and the promotion of healthy connective tissues. Vitamin C is a classic antioxidant and its use has been associated with the prevention and treatment of a variety of chronic diseases, including cardiovascular disease. Vitamin C is destroyed by excessive cooking and its level is diminished in stored or preserved vegetables and fruits. An enormous amount of literature exists on the health-giving benefits of vitamin C which has been identified by some authorities as a nutrient with almost a panacea benefit for many chronic diseases. Recent research has questioned the use of large amounts of vitamin C (greater than 3 grams/day), without balancing its effects with other antioxidants. In summary, a basic knowledge of the actions of vitamins is very valuable for individuals who may skip certain foods as part of a calorie controlled diet.

## Fat in the Combat Syndrome X Diet

The selection of the ideal fat composition of a diet is an extraordinarily complex subject. In general, saturated fatty acids will tend to promote atheroma, whereas monounsaturated fats and polyunsaturated fats are not atherogenic (an oversimplification). When a polyunsaturated fat is hydrogenated, as occurs during common food processing (e.g. margarine), it becomes atherogenic, just like a saturated fat. The dietary incorporation of polyunsaturated or monounsaturated fats in preference to saturated fat is highly advantageous in Syndrome X for decreasing blood lipids and cardiovascular risk. In general, polyunsaturated fatty acids are much less effective in lowering serum cholesterol than saturated fats are at raising blood cholesterol. A notable exception are the health giving omega 3 fatty acids (found in fish oil) which have a special role in Syndrome X (vide infra).

The importance of food selection and preparation in maintaining normal blood lipids requires emphasis. Some studies have shown a link between hydrogenated fats and atherosclerosis, implying that vegetable shortenings, margarine and other hardened fats (trans-fatty acids) are to be avoided. Indeed, several studies have shown that hydrogenated polyunsaturated fats may actually elevate blood cholesterol. This has been a big question that has been posed to the margarine industry.

The cholesterol-elevating effects of some hydrogenated vegetable oils is not completely understood, but it may be related to their content of trans-fatty acids. The most plausible explanation of this phenomenon is that the trans-fatty acids that are found in processed vegetable oils have an antagonistic effect on the action of essential fatty acids. Several scientists have studied the concentration of trans-fatty acids in the fat tissue of individuals who died from coronary artery disease and they have found that the accumulation of trans-fatty acids appeared to be correlated with a risk of death. Thus, hydrogenated vegetable oil products may not be entirely safe, but they are the basis of much "junk food".

Having recognized that some fats are healthy, it should be appreciated that frying and overheating of unsaturated fats can make "good fats" into "bad fats". Oxidation of fats tends to promote their atherogenic potential and deep fried foods are notoriously high in cholesterol. The heating of cholesterol during frying results in the oxidation of cholesterol. Oxidized cholesterol is known to be toxic to arterial smooth muscle and it may promote atherosclerosis (see Section 8).

## An Overview of Obesity

It is generally correct to state that: "individuals who eat too much will tend to be overweight and those who do not eat enough will tend to be underweight". These general principles are forgotten by at least 60 percent of the United States population who are overweight and a small percentage of the population who are underweight by conventional definitions. Weight control and obesity management are among the largest industries in North America, and it is estimated that about one-quarter of the population expend about $30 billion on weight control aids in one year. A large proportion of this one quarter of the population have Syndrome X and most do not know it! Approximately 20 percent of the population are on some form of diet continuously, and three -quarters of all mid-teen girls try to lose weight. The causes of obesity are often complex, but usually involve overeating combined with some type of emotional or behavioral "disturbance" in individuals who are prone to obesity. The maintenance of psychological well-being during weight control efforts has been grossly neglected in many weight loss recommendations. Several identified causes of obesity are shown in Table 19. Being fat will "break your heart" at some stage and it is a cardinal component of Syndrome X.

| | |
|---|---|
| · Social gluttons (USA) | Medical Causes |
| · Familial predisposition | 1. Drugs |
| · Genetic obesity | 2. Surgery |
| · Diet composition | 3. Brain disease |
| · Eating patterns | 4. Endocrine causes |
| · Emotional factors | 5. Abnormal metabolism |
| | 6. INSULIN RESISTANCE |

**Table 19:** Recognized Causes of Obesity. The most common forms of obesity is "simple obesity" that is a lifestyle disorder. Insulin resistance is capitalized because it is a much more important and common cause of obesity than previously supposed.

Obesity is not always a disease of failure of self-discipline with diet or eating patterns. Often, it is not clear what the precise problem is in the causation of obesity in many individuals, except the common knowledge that "excess" calorie intake almost always occurs in their diet. This excess calorie intake is often denied and associated with inadequate energy expenditure by the body. Overeating and a sedentary lifestyle may go hand in hand to tip the balance toward being overweight and this can trigger Syndrome X.

One popular theory of obesity is the so-called "body-weight-set-point-theory". This theory implies that the body sets itself at a level in terms of weight and composition that is somewhat defended from change. The issue then becomes a consideration of the degree of defense the body exerts to change. For example, this theory promotes the notion that obese individuals have a "high set point" and will tend to resist weight loss when placed on a low-calorie diet. Clearly, this notion is simplistic and probably only partially correct. The body-weight-set-point theory affords an important argument against the "lack of self-discipline concepts" that can defeat an obese individual's desire to want to change their body. The psychology of weight control is highly complex. It involves guilt, denial, projection and rationalizations for many – a circumstance also encountered in "addictive behavior".

## MEASURING WEIGHT STATUS

There is an important and often overlooked issue in the management of obesity, namely, the distinction between being "obese" and being "overweight". The concept of "ideal" body weight is unfortunate, but it does provide a useful, crude reference point for determining a definition of being overweight or obese. There is no ideal body weight per se but an "ideal body weight range", which takes into account differences in age, body type, and other variables. There are many standard tables to define ideal or desirable body weight, but they do not often make important allowances for the variables mentioned. The underlying importance of defining desirable body weight is really to identify a range of weight where the occurrence of diseases, caused by being overweight, are at their lowest.

The process of assessing desirable weight can be made very complex by the application of mathematical formulae. A useful and simple measure of assessment of obesity is the body mass index (BMI), which is essentially the relationship between height and weight. The BMI is calculated by dividing a person's weight in kilograms by their height in meters (which has to be squared mathematically). Overweight is approximately defined as a BMI of 25 to 30 kg/m2, and obesity is a BMI above 30 kg/m2. In general, obesity is crudely defined as more than 20 % above ideal body weight, and by this definition, more than one third to one half of the population of the United States may be obese. There are one in three (33 %) Americans that have a degree of being overweight that puts them at a medical risk and many of these individuals have Syndrome X, unknowingly!

Seeking dietary advice from virtual sources such as the internet (or books) is fraught with problems. Web sites that calculate dietary needs and propose menu plans may not have a comprehensive evaluation approach. This may result in questionable nutritional advice. Slimmimg "on-line" is problematic.

## Risks and Complications of Obesity

The risks and complications of obesity are shown in Table 20. Being overweight carries a risk of premature death, but obese individuals often have other risk factors for early death, including high blood cholesterol. hypertension, coronary artery disease, renal failure, and other serious disorders. It is notable that these complications merge imperceptibly with the components and complications of Syndrome X. The complex interrelationships between the negative outcome of obesity and Syndrome X clearly fit together. One can start to understand how obesity and Syndrome X have common, adverse health consequences.

We cannot underestimate the social toll of obesity, and this is a key to understanding the defeat felt by many obese people. American and other Western societies exude constant messages about "ideal body types", which can lead to exceptional and often extreme discrimination against the obese person. Nutritionists and physicians may succumb to the jargon of ideal body weight and type. Discrimination against the obese individual is inappropriate and it does not serve the purpose of motivating the obese person to lose weight.

## Obesity and Unhappiness

The social and economic disadvantages of being obese has not received the attention it deserves in our society. The rejection of obese individuals is shocking and destructive. It is as much of a problem as is racial discrimination. Obese adults and children face real psychosocial pressures which can affect their lifestyle choices. Obesity is known to create a legacy of hurt, especially for children.

Some studies show that obesity in childhood leads to low self esteem and obese adults may be directed to lower paid jobs. It is widely recognized that weight control involves a process of positive lifestyle choices with behavior modification. The unhappiness associated with obesity may often create a vicious cycle of self defeating behavior that impairs an individuals ability to control weight. Weight control tactics do not result in triumph without optimism. This reinforces the need to apply the very important principal of behavior modification for sustained weight control. Obese individuals often have "brain lock" of behavior that must be unlocked (see Section 6, Lifestyle to combat Syndrome X).

- Glucose intolerance
- Diabetes mellitus
- Hypertension
- Hypercholesterolemia
- Cardiac disease: atherosclerotic disease, congestive heart failure
- Pulmonary disease: sleep apnea, chronic lung disease
- Cerebrovascular disease, stroke
- Social problems:
- Cancer: breast, uterus, colon, prostate
- Gallbladder stones
- Pregnancy risks
- Surgery risks
- Renal failure
- Gout
- Infertility
- Degenerative arthritis
- Early death
- Psychological problems: poor self-image discrimination in jobs, education, and marriage

**Table 24:** Risks and Complications of Obesity. All of these problems can be encountered in Syndrome X (Syndrome X, Y and Z... is now further supported as a concept).

## CAUTIONS FOR THE DIETER

Being too fat (or too thin) is clearly dangerous to an individual's health. Incidentally, so is having a cholesterol that is too high or too low or having hypertension(see Section 2). The obese individual places more mechanical stress on their heart and body than the person of normal body weight. One seldom encounters a mature, grossly-obese, adult patient who does not have arthritis or pain in weight bearing joints. Whilst stress on joints may be obvious, the stress on the heart may not be immediately apparent. If any individual is very fat, has obesity dating back to childhood, or has adverse medical consequences of obesity, they should seek supervision and advice from healthcare giver to select optimum weight control tactics. However, not all physicians or givers of natural health care have great experience or knowledge of the treatment of severe states of obesity, so the healthcare seeker is advised to choose their counsel wisely. Bear in mind that treating obesity is a multi-billion dollar industry that is laden with quacks and quick-fix methods of weight loss. I recommend highly that readers take a look at the book "The Fat of the Land". This book is an example of  truthful investigative reporting that told consumers what they did not what to hear about weight loss tactics, causing it to have modest sales. I am willing to risk the same fate!

## Eating Disorders May be Forgotten

Before an individual decides to diet, they should assess their body habitus and decide if they fall into a category of being over-weight. This sounds so obvious that a reader may question: "Why this is worthy of mention?" The reason is that "eating disorders" result in weight status ranging from a body habitus of emaciation to the grossly obese. Eating disorders may cause problems that are more serious than simple obesity itself. Indeed, eating disorders are sometimes much more life threatening than obesity per se. Young women with anorexia nervosa may start out as "mildly chubby" teenagers.

It has been suggested that eating disorders are more common among females, especially in the 15 to 30 year age group. The estimations of the prevalence of eating disorders in this age group may shock the uninformed. With variable expression of severity, up to one-third of all females aged 15-30 years may have an atypical eating disorder, up to 1 in 20 may have bulimia nervosa, 1 in 100 may have anorexia nervosa, whereas, about 2 in 20 (or more) are obese.

Exact information on the occurrence of eating disorders is very difficult to estimate because the afflicted do not readily disclose their problem and they do not often respond with fidelity to common survey methods. The major characteristics of common eating disorders are summarized in Table 25. Many purveyors of dietary advice forget the importance of spotting the "inappropriate dieter". Catastrophes can ensue from assisting the bulimic or anorexic to lose weight! Current fad diets do not always consider these important public health issues and people with eating disorders are apt to select extreme methods of weight loss. Eating disorders  can be a more immediate threat to life than cardiovascular disabilities and they may themselves cause cardiovascular disease. Certainly, many fad diets can be predicted to cause problems in the individual with Syndrome X.

| Disorder | Main Characteristics |
|---|---|
| Anorexia Nervosa | - Morbid fear of becoming fat<br>- Marked loss of weight<br>- Amenorrhoea<br>- Not due necessarily to organic or psychiatric disease, but may be accompanied by such disease<br>- BMI 15 or less, 75% of actual body weight<br>- Unusual weight loss habits |
| Bulimia Nervosa | - Compulsive binge eating<br>- Many features in common with anorexia nervosa<br>- Binge more than twice per week for at least three months<br>- Lack of control or severe dependence on eating<br>- Regularly engage in strict weight loss regimens<br>- Persistent concern with body shape and weight |
| Atypical Eating Disorders | - Eating disorders otherwise not specified<br>- Chaotic eating patterns<br>- May have many, but not all of the diagnostic criteria of anorexia or bulimia nervosa<br>- May be recovering from or transitioning toward anorexia and bulimia |
| Obesity | - May or may not be an eating disorder per se<br>- Very heterogeneous components |

- Has genetic, organic,
  psychological and nutritional
  potential of origin
- Severe obesity usually has a
  well-developed psychological
  component

**Table 25:** The characteristics of the main four types of eating disorders are summarized. Recognition of these features in an individual should result in seeking medical advice. Eating disorders are potentially life threatening.

## MORE ABOUT OBESITY AND HEALTH

The health consequences of obesity are a matter for major concern as we recognize obesity as the commonest consequence of "malnutrition" in developed countries. The US has engaged in a form of "nutritional colonialsim" with "fast food" which may be endangering the health of underdeveloped countries. Much research has attempted to predict the forms of obesity that create the greatest risks. In general, it is excess body fat, located in the organs of the body (visceral obesity), that presents an independent risk factor for cardiovascular disease and many other diseases. The accumulation of excessive body fat leads to insulin resistance which then results in the high blood sugar, insulin, cholesterol and blood pressure which so typifies the killer constellation of Syndrome X. If we set Syndrome X aside, the illnesses that are well documented to be associated with obesity create a formidable list (Table 26).

| High Risk | Moderate Risk | Lower Risk |
|---|---|---|
| Diabetes Mellitus | Heart disease | Cancer of womb, breast, colon |
| Insulin Resistance | Peripheral vascular disease | Hormonal disorders, especially sex hormones |
| Hypertension | Stroke | Infertility |

| | | |
|---|---|---|
| High blood fats | Arthritis, both osteoarthritis and gout | Congenital defects in children of obese mothers |
| Gallstones | Polycystic Ovary Syndrome | Increased accident rates |
| Sleep apnea | Low back pain | Depression |
| Decreased aerobic fitness potential | Fibromyalgia Medical risk in surgery | Social isolation |

**Table 26:** Illnesses definitely associated with being overweight. Risks for these diseases tends to increase by degrees of obesity which can be measured by methods such as the calculation of body mass index (BMI). Note: Overlap of risk exists for each disease or disorder in the spectrum of being obese ("degrees of fatness") and the first four factors in the high risk column relate to Syndrome X.

## CRITICAL ELEMENTS OF DIETS

Critical elements in the management of obesity are "diet" with reduced calorie (restricted simple sugar and saturated fat intake), nutrition education, and behavioral modification techniques. It is recognized that refined sugar and saturated fat in the diet of Western society is a pivotal element in promoting obesity. Many nutritional surveys have shown that Western populations have changed their diets over the past century to increase calorie intake from saturated fat, while decreasing the dietary intake of calories derived from complex carbohydrates found in fruit and vegetables. It is significant to note that if calorie intake is kept the same, a diet rich in fat will, almost always, produce enhanced gain of body fat. This finding is well documented in animal and human experiments and it proposes a clear reason to reject the liberal saturated-fat approach to dieting (e.g. Atkin's Diet), at least for any long term use. I acknowledge that the Atkins' Diet and similar diet plans have emerged with a new label as a form of "low carb lifestyle" that may have merits in Syndrome X and the value of healthy fats (omega 3 fatty acids) is now proposed by Dr. Robert

Atkins and others. However, these issues are not very clear in the "New or Old Atkins' Diet Revolution".

Routine medical treatment of obesity using diet alone has a failure rate of greater than 95 percent over a 3 year period. In addition, the practice of drastic calorie reduction is known to be associated with a "YoYo" pattern of weight loss and rebound weight gain. I believe that rebound weight gain is a common problem following the induction of dietary ketosis that occurs with liberal fat intake and strict carbohydrate restriction. It has been documented that both men and women whom reduce their calorie intake below 1200 calories per day and then resume prior dietary patterns may enter into a process of even increasing weight gain over time. This may be explained by the downwards correction of body metabolism that occurs to accommodate to low-calorie intake. This downwards compensation of body metabolism which occurs as a consequence of calorie restriction does not rapidly reverse. Thus, the reinstitution of normal eating could promote weight gain in the individual with an acquired (diet-induced) down-regulation of body metabolism. Exercise and behavior modification can help to break the "Yo Yo" effect.

## DIFFERENT DIRECTIONS WITH DIETS

There are several different types of dietary approaches to weight loss (Table 27). Individuals who have tried the "Zone", "Sugar Busters" etc., can recognize how they fit into a dietary direction of altered macronutrient intake (fat, carbohydrate and protein), but the direction is not always self-recognized. Most popular diets unfortunately fit the "fad" classification. Each general dietary approach listed in Table 26 has disadvantages or limitations, underscoring the need for the healthcare professional and the patient to consider a more holistic and tailored approach to weight control. The basis of what I consider to be a holistic approach must focus on education in nutrition. This approach should include at least a consideration of the following: a healthy calorie-controlled diet, nutrition-education, behavioral therapy, exercise therapy, and motivational interventions with training in "dietary" compliance.

| Diet Type | Disadvantages |
|---|---|
| Balanced low-calorie diet* | Hunger, preoccupation with food and frequent failure. |
| Formula diets | The discipline of the diet creates boredom and failure, and formulas are expensive. |
| Specific nutrient addition | Higher fiber is the frequent choice, but palatability is a problem; worthy of more study. |
| Specific nutrient elimination | Specific nutrient deficiency syndromes, special preparation, poor compliance. |
| Fad diets | Sometimes dangerous, often expensive, usually a variation of one or more of the above options. |

**Table 27:** Commonly used types of diet for weight loss or obesity management. (*) Balanced low-calorie diets with soluble fiber (beta glucan) and foods with a low glycemic index that are presented creatively with other lifestyle adjustments are the best option. Weight loss must be healthy.

The importance of inducing a long-term change in behavior in eating habits must be stressed again; and the individual undergoing a weight control program should be aware of the risks of continued obesity and understand that the optimal approach is a long-term strategy. Drug therapy for obesity has been used as a useful adjunct to management in some patients, but amphetamine-like drugs or Ephedra containing supplements (Ma Huang) are best avoided, even though they may be effective in the short-term. These drugs and supplements can make Syndrome X worse, at least by raising blood pressure. Whilst these supplements are "energizing", the loss of energy in Syndrome X is due to poor use of sugar by the body. This cannot be corrected by "energizing supplements", it has to be addressed by tackling insulin resistance and glucose intolerance. Drug therapy for obesity, if used, should be only a short-term approach in selected patients.

## FURTHER DISPELLING THE FADS: LOOKING AT DIETS

All diets could be considered an attempt at self-imposed, distorted eating patterns. Unfortunately, good eating patterns are harder to achieve than bad eating patterns. I reiterate that the recommendation of so many different diets is sure proof that none are entirely effective for tackling weight control in a sustained (or healthy) manner. It is not possible within the remit of this book to give an intricate account of the pros and cons of each diet, except to say that most weight reducing diets are designed for weight loss alone, sometimes at the expense of the lack of promotion of cardiovascular wellness, and often at the expense of not combating Syndrome X. Weight loss is often an important component of achieving cardiovascular wellness, but some weight reduction strategies are to be avoided in the cardiac patient. Again, the reader is advised to check with a healthcare practitioner. A little knowledge or an "old wives" (or "old husbands") reassurance can be dangerous to health and longevity.

The "balanced diet" is the optimal choice for weight control, since this selection helps control hunger, is not monotonous and it improves overall health. Understanding why a particular diet was developed can assist in matching dietary interventions for changing needs. For example, initial strict weight reducing diets should be time dependent and a maintenance diet that is more relaxed can be introduced subsequently to control weight or prevent weight gain. Certain diets can improve overall health or correct existing disease when they are tailored to the individuals' needs. A number of diets contain very specific meal recommendations. This degree of regimentation is preferred by some, but complied with by few. The normal mode or pace of life in Western society makes it very difficult to comply with a specifically regimented diet. If an individual does not choose a diet option that matches their lifestyle to some degree, failure will be inevitable!

Certain diets are recommended by institutions or organizations that have an aura of authority in their espoused opinions. Many scientists and authors agree that because a diet is promoted by a government or institution of high standing then it does not necessarily mean that the dietary recommendations are ideal. Some organizations have "axes to grind" or receive support from industrial sources that may "color" their recommendations. Table 28 summarizes two general diet proposals from conventional bodies of opinion. These diets have some advantages, but they also possess disadvantages or limitations, especially when it comes to combat against the killer constellation of Syndrome X.

| Diet/Characteristics | Comments |
|---|---|
| The American Heart Association Diet (Less saturated fat, low salt, more complex carbohydrates) | - Easy to follow<br>- Widespread medical use<br>- Evidence it may prevent heart disease<br>- Omits the importance of essential fat in cardiovascular disease prevention or treatment<br>- Some choices of polyunsaturated fat sources are suspect<br>- Forgot the role of soluble fiber, soy and vegetable protein<br>- Does not directly address Syndrome X |
| The U.S. Dept. of Agriculture Dietary Recommendations (Pyramid of Foods) | - Aimed at general health promotion but it fails in places<br>- Does not consider importance of essential fatty acids |

- Too accepting of
  processed foods
- No real focus of the
  health benefit
- Does not address refined
  sugars or Syndrome X

**Table 28:** Some potential drawbacks of well accepted health giving diets. Both of these proposals do not address insulin resistance or Syndrome X, per se.

Some of the more "popular" diets that have gained "commercial" acceptance are summarized in Table 29. In many cases, the medical profession, both of the "conventional" and "alternative" persuasion, have rejected these diets, for one reason or another, in favor of more balanced and optimal nutrition. Like most things in life, it is generally the extremes that are dangerous. Optimization of food intake is often synonymous with moderation. Claims that you can eat what you like and lose weight are very misleading, often to the point of being frankly untrue. "Eat what you want and lose weight", "eat yourself thin", "all you can eat to lose weight" etc. are nonsensical statements that sell books.

| Diet/Description | Criticisms: Valid or Otherwise? |
|---|---|
| Dr. Atkins Diet Revolution (high fat, high protein, low carbohydrates) (Banting Diet, Taller's Diet Harvey's Diet) | - Not a revolution, used by William Banting in the 1800's and intermittently in 20th century<br>- Accelerated early weight loss is water loss<br>- May result in abnormal blood lipids<br>- YoYo regain of weight can occur<br>- Ketosis induced with potential negative metabolic consequences |

|  | - Cannot be recommended for the person with cardiovascular disease |
|  | - Uncontrolled, unhealthy fat intake causes cardiovascular disease |
| Dr. Stillman's Quick Inches Off Diet (low protein, high carbohydrates) | - Few merits<br>- Modification of 1950's Rice Diet<br>- Accelerated early weight loss is water loss<br>- YoYo regain of weight can occur<br>- Nutritionally deficient<br>- Dangerous in Syndrome X |
| The Zen Macrobiotic Diet and other macrobiotic diet (grain based vegetarian diet) | - Nutritionally incomplete<br>- Not recommended long-term because of dangers of nutrient depletion<br>- Beyond the average reach of compliance<br>- Lack of certain essential fatty acids<br>- Very variable dietary formu lations that are complex with a questionable basis |
| The Living Foods Diet (Based on uncooked organic vegetables) | - Ecological sense<br>- Stresses inclusion of vegeta bles over grains in contrast to many macrobiotic diets<br>- More to do with food prepa ration<br>- Probably healthy and is good for partial incorporation into a dietary regimen<br>- Only for the very committed |

Weight Watchers
(well established plan for
weight reduction)

- Quite successful
- Shortcomings in the control
  of blood cholesterol and
  hypertension
- Expensive
- Forgot fiber, essential fats
  and soy
- Advantage of group support

The New American Diet
(dietary transition program
traditional American diet to a
more 'vegetarian' diet that is
high in complex carbohydrates
and low in saturated fats)

- Much to commend this diet
- Well-balanced and flexible
- Good accompanying manual
- Recognizes omega 3 benefits,
  underestimates omega 6 benefits
- Forgot to emphasize fiber
  and vegetable protein.

The Beverly Hills Diet or
The Fit for Life Diet
(Emphasizes fruit intake)

- The notion that fruit melts
  fat is not valid
- Causes diarrhea
- May gain weight
- Not popular in Beverly Hills

The Pritikin Program
(Quite severe diet restrictions
with cardiovascular wellness
potential of low fat, low
cholesterol)

- Compliance problems
- Nutritionally incomplete
- Not advised for Syndrome X
- Has some valid basis

The Dolly Parton Diet
('Prescribed' diet with
on/off eating)

- Little, if any, scientific basis
- Food juggling regimen is too
  complex

The Dean Ornish Program
(A complete lifestyle program
with low cholesterol objective
for cardiovascular wellness)

- Very sound program that has
  been subjected to objective
  research
- Compliance problems
- Great support plan
- Behavior modification strong

| | |
|---|---|
| The Scarsdale Diet (Short-term ketosis induction plan) | - Dangerous without medical supervision<br>- Use for only 2 weeks advised<br>- Loss of protein tissue (muscle) occurs<br>- Rejected by many as a fad |
| The Last Chance Diet (Liquid protein diet) | - Short-term<br>- Risk of sudden death<br>- Thrown out by many |
| Fasting is a Way of Life (Essentially, just don't eat) | - Prolonged fasts are decidedly dangerous<br>- Boring<br>- Stimulates overeating |
| The Cambridge Diet or The Slim-Fast Plan (Beverage assisted weight loss) | - Monotonous<br>- No education on eating properly<br>- Not nutritionally complete meal replacements<br>- Compliance problems<br>- Short-term success only |
| The Set Point Diet (Based on the theory that everyone has a set point (weight point) which the body fights to maintain) | - Balanced with natural foods<br>- Similar to AHA and USDA<br>- No emphasis on essential fatty acids<br>- Principal aim weight loss<br>- A good start |
| The Zone Diet | - Much to commend this approach<br>- Engages the issues of Syndrome X<br>- Too much protein? |

| Reaven's Diet (and variations) | - Highly commendable for Syndrome X (see text)<br>- The way to go with a tailored, "back to basics" approach<br>- Outcome research not avail able |
|---|---|

**Table 29:** This table contains some subjective comments based on a study of the diets by the author and consultations with medical practitioners and patients who have experiences. Some of the commonly used diet programs are listed with putative or actual concerns about their application. With exception of the AHA and Ornish Programs, the other dietary methodologies have been somewhat lacking in careful clinical study. Assessments of their safety and efficacy have been anecdotal. This situation may make criticisms of the diet plans appear anecodotal, so the author has focused on his medical interpretations of the basis, if any, for the dietary interventions.

## OBESITY: A COMBINATION OF FACTORS

Obesity is caused by a complex interaction between an individuals genetic tendency to weight gain and environmental issues. A person is most likely to become fat when their hereditary tendency to develop obesity is combined with psycho-social influences that may contribute to weight gain. The relative contribution of genetic tendencies or environmental tendencies to obesity in the process of weight gain varies considerably from person to person. The state of being fat is a heterogeneous disorder (many different manifestations and causes). This situation helps to explain why no single approach to weight control e.g. drug treatment or specific diet can be expected to be universally successful. Approaches to weight control need to be tailored to the individuals' needs.

## MANAGING WEIGHT CONTROL

The ideas that there is a simple set of dietary guidelines or an easy way to control weight gain or cause weight loss are best put to rest. Whilst many individuals crave weight loss and the attainment of an "ideal" body weight, many studies show us that this circumstance is rarely achieved. Therefore, the objectives of a weight control program should be clear. These objectives may include minor, moderate or great degrees of weight loss, but for many people it involves a desire to maintain an existing body weight (weight control).

Failures of weight loss programs are "written in the stars" when the stated objectives are unattainable. It is now apparent that a reduction in body weight for the obese by a factor of 10% is a reasonable short term goal (over months). I believe that "baby steps" are likely to be more successful in the long term than "crash diets" or other drastic weight loss attempts. Losing 10 to 15 % of body weight for the moderately or severe obese person is a good platform to attempt the goal of approaching a "normal weight". Recent studies show that modest weight loss can make a real difference in the prevention of diabetes mellitus and the components of Syndrome X.

## REITERATING THE ABSENCE OF THE IDEAL DIET

We have learned that the concept of the "ideal" diet is like the concept of "ideal" weight – it is wishful thinking. Let's ask some questions. Why are there so many diets? Why do diet books sell well? Which is the best diet? Attempts to answer these questions start to form the basis of a rational approach to weight loss. There are so many diets because no single diet is ideal for everyone. The persistent but erroneous belief that there may be an ideal diet leads to a constant search for the right diet. This desperate quest is reinforced by the lack of success of an individual diet. The principal problem with weight loss diets is that they only have weight loss in mind, not the promotion of health. Furthermore, short term weight loss is often achieved by "diets," but studies show that only 5% of individuals can maintain significant weight loss over a 5 year period.

"Just" as "just" lowering cholesterol or "just" controlling blood pressure are not worthy objectives, "just" losing weight is a misguided approach. The best approach achieves the weight control objective, whilst dealing with other important health issues. Nowhere is this approach more important than in the combat against Syndrome X (or Syndrome X, Y and Z...), where a constellation of disorders requires correction. In other words, a calorie controlled weight loss program may not overcome insulin resistance and its consequences (Syndrome X), if the selection of foods in the diet is wrong. In fact, a poorly constructed diet for weight loss can be dangerous to health. Not all studies confirm that weight loss leads to automatic wellness, but well planned voluntary weight loss is associated consistently with health advantages.

## Losing Weight: The Nitty Gritty

Recent scientific symposia that attempt to reach a consensus opinion on healthy weight loss diets have led to arguments (e.g. USDA forum, 2000). Indeed, each proposed "popular" dietary approach possesses disadvantages and limitations for portability. This situation must make us take a step backwards and examine the principles of healthy weight control and apply them. I repeat that we have reached a point where it must be "back to basics" before we can move forward. Winston Churchill, who battled obesity, stated "the farther you look back, the further forward you can go", even though he was not referring to corpulence.

It is very important to realize that losing weight should not result in loss of lean body mass (muscle); it should be aimed at gaining muscle, whilst shedding fat. Thus, weight control involves a careful consideration of the retention of an ideal body composition which, in simple terms, means a healthy muscle to fat ratio in the body. The health consequences of building muscle mass during weight control have been underestimated in many weight-loss guidelines.

Predictably, the retention of an ideal body composition involves exercise, as well as balanced nutrition. Despite any claims to the contrary, the most effective way to lose weight or prevent weight gain is calorie restriction or control in the diet combined with exercise. This "back to basics" discussion of weight control is supported by the vital role that a healthy functioning muscle mass plays in burning energy (taking up glucose), promoting insulin sensitivity and enhancing the body's oxidative capacity.

If muscle mass is lost, then aerobic capacity of the body is reduced, less sugar is utilized by muscle, or stored as glycogen, and more of the energy intake in the diet (carbohydrate or fat) is stored as fat. This latter process is called lipogenesis (fat creation) and it tends to occur with aging where less glucose is transferred into muscles or less muscle is available to accept the glucose. It has been underestimated that greater one in four men and one in three women will have an abnormal glucose tolerance when they reach the age of seventy years and this is related to increases in the body fat content compared with muscle content, together with the emergence of insulin insensitivity. A combat against Syndrome X must involve support to build muscle structure and function.

In summary, the function of the body's muscle mass is highly relevant to Syndrome X. The muscles of the body are the principal site of glucose uptake and when exercise occurs the muscles burn up dietary glucose and insulins' actions are promoted. The greater the amount and efficiency of muscle activity, the more glycogen becomes stored in muscle to provide an energy reserve for subsequent exercise. In contrast, people with a low muscle mass who are sedentary have a circumstance where lipogenesis (fat accumulation) in the body tends to occur. These are reasons why people with Syndrome X protest their lack of energy and slothful life.

## RECOMMENDATIONS ON DIET PLANS

First and foremost, I do not recommend that an individual think in dietary terms only for weight loss, but rather consider an overall plan for lifestyle adjustment (Table 30). We have learned that diets are impositions or deviations of "normal" (in many people normal is abnormal) eating patterns and habits. The term habit is important because without motivation and considerable behavior modification all diets will fail. The literature on behavioral change in relationship to eating is voluminous, but changing behavior is difficult, especially when our society reinforces the status quo. The issues can be summarized as getting to know yourself, recognize your tricks and catch yourself with a change (see Section 6, Lifestyle to Combat Syndrome X). Weight control is often a process of self-identification of the problem and self-intervention.

- Maintain an optimal weight
- Control elevated blood pressure
- Engage in physical activity
- Do not smoke or inhale second hand smoke
- Reduce your dietary intake of saturated fat and cholesterol, select vegetable protein
- Pay special attention to your mind and psychological well-being
- Do not use dietary supplements as a way of supplementing a lousy diet
- Remember the mirror life: your imput is your return
- Moderation in most pleasures is advisable
- Use natural substances to promote cardiovascular well-being e.g. soluble fiber, soy, fish oil
- Conventional medicine when used appropriately has advantages
- Consider the possible presence of Syndrome X

**Table 30:** An overall lifestyle plan must accompany a diet for health. Weight control is a function of calorie control, exercise and behavior modification for most people.

| Dietary Maneuver | Health Outcome | |
|---|---|---|
| | Prevents Heart Disease | Treats Heart Disease |
| * Incorporate soluble fiber especially beta glucan soluble fiber fractions | Yes (x, z, y) | Yes (x, z, y) |
| * Incorporate balanced omega 3 and omega 6 fatty acids in diet | Yes (x, z, y) | Yes (x, z, y) |
| Add soy protein | Yes (x, z) | Yes (x, z) |
| Lower calorie intake | Yes (y) | Yes (y) |
| Lower cholesterol intake | Yes (x) | Yes (x) |
| * Lower saturated fat intake | Yes (x) | Yes (x) |

| | | |
|---|---|---|
| * Lower salt intake | Yes (y) | Yes (y) |
| Switch from animal to vegetable protein, e.g. soy | Yes (x, z) | Yes (x) |
| * Move from simple to complex carbohydrate sources | Yes (x) | Yes (x) |
| Lower alcohol intake | Yes (x, z, y) | Yes (x, z, y) |

**Table 31:** Dietary changes that both prevent and treat heart disease directly and indirectly. NOTE: (x) signifies lowers cholesterol; (z) signifies beneficial cardiovascular effects independent of lowering cholesterol; and (y) = signifies direct or indirect effect on lowering blood pressure. The asterisk (*) denotes particular value in Syndrome X, but all of the interventions can help combat Syndrome X.

The most important aspect of diet planning is to set objectives and goals. The individual must understand why they want to diet. What is the need? — defined by the presence or absence of a disease status or a global health initiative or requirement. No single diet can be given as a panacea recommendation, as indicated by the previous review of the many existing dietary recommendations. The important concept is that various meals work towards different health outcomes. In the absence of sufficient individual knowledge concerning the health potential of various foods, a rational dietary program cannot be constructed. Table 31 summarizes how certain selected dietary interventions may work in cardiovascular disease prevention or treatment. Note the multiple benefits, direct or indirect, that simple dietary changes may make on cardiovascular wellness.

## The "Slow Food" Movement

We (Americans) are apparently blessed with a fast food restaurant on every urban street. Whilst everyone is "on the go", the quick burger and fries is too convenient and inexpensive to avoid. Fast food caters to our "fat and sweet" taste-preferences and most of the food is high in saturated fat, salt, refined (simple) sugars and low in dietary fiber. In addition, burgers, fries and break-fast sandwiches can be "wolfed down" in a manner that provides "fleeting" pleasure.

Aside from the unhealthy composition of fast food, eating under hurried or stressed conditions has been shown to cause higher blood cholesterol and it often precipitates unpleasant digestive symptoms. Eating under stress can cause spikes in LDL cholesterol and blood triglycerides. In addtion, rapid distension of the stomach with carbohydrates promotes rapid emptying of the stomach, rapid absorption of sugar and increases in insulin secretion. This promotes glucose intolerance, insulin resistance and worsens Syndrome X. High blood sugar followed by rapid surges in blood insulin can cause "overswings" in blood sugar control resulting in a tendency to experience reactive hypoglycemia (low blood sugar)and cravings.

I believe that these circumstances can promote obesity and contribute to the components of Syndrome X. Furthermore, rapid swings in blood sugar can cause mood and behavioral changes in adults and children who are particularly susceptible to "sugar highs" (and "lows"). Craving or seeking the highs is a common phenomenon which is really and example of "food addiction". Just how much damage results from eating under stress in a hurried manner is speculative, but it does cause medical and sociobehavioral problems. Meals are best enjoyed in a ceremonious, relaxed manner as part of the "slow food movement." Making time for oneself is a key issue in the combat against Syndrome X.

## "Feeling Full" for Weight Loss

The promotion of a sensation of feeling full with meals that do not deliver a large amount of calories is a very valuable maneuver for weight control. This perception of being full is a signal sent from the gastrointestinal tract, especially the stomach, to the brain and it causes a sensation of "satisfaction" or "satiety". Anything that stretches the stomach can cause an activation of "stretch receptors" in the wall of the stomach. This alerts the brain to the idea that enough has been eaten. Whilst scientists have attempted to unravel the mechanisms of the promotion of satiety, the presence of stretch receptors in the stomach that trigger complex neurohormonal events (mind-body connections) were discovered and characterized more than thirty years ago by veterinary scientists (Iggo receptors).

The most important way to use this simple and safe "satiety trick" is to choose foods that are low in calories (low calorie density). The obvious choice is dietary fiber where bulk is given without significant calorie intake (see Section 7, The Secret of Soluble Fiber). This effect is most notable with fractions of soluble fiber (e.g. beta glucan) that causes a viscous, bulky suspension that both stretches the stomach and has a further advantage of delaying the rate at which the stomach empties its contents into the small bowel. Soluble fiber fractions (e.g. beta glucan glucocolloids) are the ultimate low caloric density foods with low glycemic indices.

Caloric density of food is a useful measure to consider if one is going to use the "satiety promoting (feel full) weight loss method". It can be calculated easily for many foods by dividing a foods' calories by its weight in grams. Thinking about these simple mathematics is quite easy and the most important objective is to choose a food with low caloric density. Carbohydrates and proteins provide 5 calories per gram, whereas fat gives 9 calories per gram. Using the simple calculation, 100 grams of butter gives 900 calories and it has a calorie density of 900 divided by 100 i.e. a caloric density of 9 which is very high in comparison with plain yogurt that has a caloric density of approximately 1.5. Table 32 gives examples of the caloric density of various foods. Choosing foods with a low caloric density and low glycemic index in a balanced manner is often rewarded by safe weight control.

---

### The "Feel Full Weight Loss Trick" involves:

- **Food of low caloric density**
- **Food of low glycemic index**

**It is a safe weight control tactic**

**See: Syndrome X Nutritional Factors (Section 8)**

## CALORIC DENSITY OF SOME FOOD, QUOTED IN A RANGE

| Low | Moderate | High |
|---|---|---|
| Water 0 | Pasta 1.4-2.0 | Butter 7-9 |
| Diet drinks <0.1 | Cheese 2.6-4.0 | Margarine 4-8 |
| Soluble fiber <0.1 | French Fries 3.5-4.0 | Nuts 6.0-7.0 |
| Many beans 0.6-0.8 | Regular salad | Chocolate 5-5.5 |
| Vegetables 0.15-1.1 | Dressings 3.5-6.0 | Potato or corn chips |
| Salads 0.12-1.0 | Fish 0.9-2.0 | 4.7-6 Red meat |
| | Skinless chicken 0.9-1.8 | (depends on fat) 1-4 |
| | | Chicken with skin >4 |

**Table 32:** Examples of the caloric density of some common foods. Note: Soluble fiber extracts have very low caloric density and they are the ultimate form of food with a low glycemic index. Note: some foods cross over from low to moderate to high caloric density, simple sugars are to be avoided. Further Note: caloric density is not the same as glycemic index, e.g. pasta has a moderate caloric density, but when it contains refined carbohydrate it has a high glycemic index.

## NOVEL WAYS TO INDUCE SATIETY

The sensation of satiety (feeling satisfied or full) after meals involves complex neurohormonal controls. Whilst stretching the stomach and slowing the emptying rate of the stomach with soluble fiber are useful ways of inducing satiety, much interest has focused on the hormone cholecystokinin (CCK) as a principal satiety "signal" in the body. More than twenty years ago, scientists discovered that the administration of the hormone CCK could make people feel full (satiated) even without eating.

The hormone CCK is produced in response to the dietary intake of protein and certain fats. This hormone is released by an intermediary hormone called CCK-releasing peptide which can be destroyed by pancreatic enzymes that are secreted after a meal. The secretion of CCK is also interrupted by bile acid secretions from the liver and CCK causes the gallbladder to contract.

Naturals ways to enhance the output of CCK or prolong its

secretion can be used to induce a reduction in food intake in humans. Giving substances that release CCK e.g. certain proteins and fats (long chain fatty acids, e.g. oleic acid) and stop the breakdown of the CCK-releasing peptide e.g. enzyme inhibitors from soy or root crops (potatos) may induce prolonged satiety. This approach complements the action of soluble fiber on inducing the "feel-full-weight-loss-trick". Examples of these natural products are marketed as Satiety Factors™ and Satietrol™ and they are valuable as adjuncts to weight control.

## Drug and Supplements for Weight

Whilst weight control depends on the basic issues of caloric control, exercise, behavior modification and lifestyle change, many individuals seek adjunctive help to shed pounds. I see nothing wrong with this extra help, if these weight loss adjuncts are chosen with wisdom. Drugs and dietary supplements can form a reasonable "back up" plan for weight loss but the disadvantages of their use requires recognition. Table 33 summarizes popular drug or dietary supplement approaches and their potential "ups and downs". I believe that many drugs and ephedrine (ephedra, Ma Huang) containing supplements are best avoided because they share a common problem of raising blood pressure. The only 'drug" that seems, at first sight, to be suitable for use as a weight loss agent is Orlistat (Xenical). This drug blocks fat absorption and it causes anal leakage, gas and diarrhoea – unattractive prospects !.

| Drugs | Comments |
|---|---|
| Fen-phen | Withdrawn for cardiovascular damage – probably caused by fenfluramine component. |
| Silbutramine (Meridia) | Loss of 10 pounds more than placebo in 12 months (modest effect), but causes headache, constipation, insomnia and high blood pressure. |
| Orlistat (Xenical) | Blocks fat absorption, but causes oily anal leakage, gas and diarrhoea. |

| Phenyl propanolamine (Dexatrim, Acutrim) | Questionable appetite suppression, but raises blood pressure. |

| **Supplements** | **Comments** |
| --- | --- |
| Ephedra (Ma Huang) (Xendrine, Diet Max) | When combined with caffeine in high dose may be effective. Raises blood pressure and associated with deaths. |
| Pyruvate | May be effective and safe but dose high, better used in a combination product. |
| Chromium (Chromax, Carnochrome) | Arguments about efficacy for weight loss alone but very advantageous in Syndrome X. |
| Chitosan | Blocks fat absorption – may be valuable and safe. |
| Conjugated linoleic (Tonalin) acid | Questionable effectiveness when used alone |
| Hydroxycitric acid (CitriMax and Citrin) | Good for combination, products questionable effectiveness when used alone. |
| DHEA (dehydroeipiand-rosterone) | A steroid "drug", may raise blood pressure –best avoided. |
| Hydrolyzed collagen (Calorad, Metrim PM etc.) | Many anecdotal reports of success, mechanism of action not clear – utililization of hydroxyproline? Reported to improve skin tone? |

**Table 33:** An overview of weight loss drugs and supplements.

When one examines weight loss drugs and supplements in terms of safety and effectiveness, no single item emerges with clear advantages. The amount of research done with drugs is much greater than that performed with supplements, but this does not mean that drugs are better. I suggest that a logical approach may be to use a "safe" combination of natural agents to act as an adjunct to diet and exercise for weight loss.

## MATCHING DIETS TO METABOLIC TYPES?

From time to time numerous suggestions are made about matching a specific diet to a "chemical status"or "body type" of an individual. There is no doubt that evolution has played a major role in our body habitus and bio-chemical functions, but efforts to match nutrition to metabolic types have been unsuccessful; perhaps because we do not know how to classify different meta-bolic types or more likely because of major interindividual and intraindivid-ual differences in body chemistry. I am suspicious of the diet to match a hypothetical biomarker or hypothesized body status. Among the most absurd of suggestions is that one can distinguish the difference between "slow burn-ers" of body fuel and "fast burners" by hair analysis.

The quest to identify a difference in metabolic types has included a look at body markers (phenotypes) such as being thin (ectomorphic), being fat (endomorphic) or being predominantly muscular (mesomorphic). However, these body types are not associated consistently with a specific "metabolic sta-tus". The body has many ways of expressing its genetic material. One simple example of gentoypic expression is blood type, and much has been made of matching diets to differences in blood groups (Type 0, A, AB, B). The evidence for this putative match of blood groups with metabolic type and specific dietary need is decidedly lacking.

The reason that simple body markers (or biomarkers) do not corre-late with metabolic status is related to the simple notion that metabolic type is determined by a "huge, mixed-bag of tricks". An endomorph can be athletic and an ectomorph can be sedentary or vice versa. One may gobble sugar whilst the other may be a vegan. Eating for a specific body type (or blood group or other "biomarker" type) is currently part of "marketing mumbo-jumbo" in the world of "dietary fads and fallacies".

## Moving Towards Meal Plans?

Meals are personal preferences. Living by someone elses' taste preferences will seldom result in a successful clinical outcome. The characteristic of a meal plan that will result in reasonable efficacy, safety and compliance is shown in Table 35. I hope that the readers may appreciate, by now, my objection to weight loss menus. Cookbooks are great resources but many physicians, including me, who discuss food choices cannot even boil an egg !

- The right diet has the right objectives for the client.
- It should provide balanced nutrition, if possible.
- The benefits should be obvious to the dieter.
- For weight loss, the diet must supply less energy than the person's energy requirements.
- When calorie intake is below 1,800 calories per day, mineral and vitamin supplements are required.
- The diet must have a high degree of acceptability. Monotony spells failure.
- It should be part of a lifestyle adjustment regimen.
- Its success is equally dependent on food exclusion and healthy food substitution.

**Table 35:** Some advantageous characteristics of a meal plan that will aid compliance and fulfill health objectives.

## Medical, Political, Social and Potential Legal Implications of Obesity

In December 2001, the Surgeon General of the US, Dr. David Satcher MD, announced that obesity was rapidly becoming the number one killer disorder in America. Obesity may be directly responsible for 300,000 deaths per year among Americans and as part of the metabolic Syndrome X, it impacts the occurrence of death from all causes. The obesity epidemic in the United States was estimated to have cost 117 billion dollars in the year 2000. The precise occurrence of obesity and overweight status among adults in the US is not known, but it is estimated to be present in more than 60% of the adult population and about 15% of children and teenagers. Please note my changing numbers, as we scramble to find the actual prevalence of obesity in the US. Arguments prevail in society concerning "the ownership" of the obesity problem. Conventional medicine has applied increasingly the "disease state model" to obesity, but sociologists and behavioral scientists have questioned this approach. Politicians have avoided addressing the obesity problem in the US, perhaps because of the massive power of "the food lobby", together with a lack of consensus about what should be done to address the problem.

There has been an increasing tendency in several Western countries for people to avoid accepting any responsibility for the choosing of adverse lifestyle. With an increasing tendency to litigation, it is now being suggested that the food industry could be held responsible for the ill health that results from being overweight. Some members of the legal profession are discussing potential legal action against several parts of the food industry because of their perceived role in causing the obesity problem. Perhaps, it is not just obesity that they should be assessing for potential litigation, but the whole issue of Syndrome X which is undoubtedly related to diet to a major degree.

I see this potential circumstance, that is similar to legal action brought against cigarette manufacturers, to be an important and emerging issue in Western society. Whilst I do not encourage anyone to blame themselves for developing obesity and its consequences, members of society have to accept responsibility for their own choices of lifestyle, including selection of their nutritional habits. Several nutritionists and medical scientists have suggested that some food companies have behaved like cigarette companies by enticing people to eat more of the wrong kind of food, in the face of knowledge that certain foods promote ill health. The obesity problem that threatens the health of the US nation is unlikely to be impacted without combined social, political and medical initiatives. Whilst attractive to some, legal action against the food industry is not likely to control the problem and US consumers may not find the consequences of this legal approach to be "palatable" in its outcome. Imagine a candy bar with a government health warning?

## Bars to Weight Control

Understanding the factors that operate to interfere with weight loss helps to create a potentially successful plan. We have learned that weight loss is often associated with an adaptation of the body where energy expenditures decrease. Furthermore, a lower body weight tends to cause lower energy requirements to maintain the weight. The body seems to work hard to maintain its weight and to cause a sustained loss of weight, an individual has to maintain a decrease in energy intake (food intake), whilst increasing expenditure by exercise. I believe that any weight loss program that is not accompanied by an exercise plan cannot lead to sustained weight control. Again, weight control requires important changes in behavior and lifestyle and these changes must be long term if weight control is required.

As part of the body's adaptations to weight loss, the ability of the person who has lost weight to burn fat for energy seems to decrease. Fat is burned by oxidation and a reduction of this process tends to cause fat taken into the diet to be stored as body fat. Whilst we shall review some of the advantages of a low carbohydrate intake for Syndrome X and weight control, those diets that recommend liberal saturated fat intake (e.g. Atkins Diet) will over the long term lead to weight gain due to a reduction of the body's ability to burn fat (oxidize fat).

I have stressed the notion that permanent changes in lifestyle and calorie intake are required to control weight. On a simple basis, it is clear that ingrained habits that may cause weight gain are hard to change, especially when they are established over a long period of time. Section 6 of this book discussed lifestyle changes and introduces the important concepts of "behavior modification". Attempts at weight control without changing behavior will fail.

Clearly, the earlier that positive lifestyle changes occur in the progression of obesity, the more likelihood of sustained success. These circumstances reinforce the need to take public health initiatives to control childhood obesity. My opinions are supported by observations that when obese parents and children attempt to control weight by working together, children appear to have a better chance to sustain weight control

I acknowledge that the reader of this book may feel bereft of "specific" direction, if certain specific recommendations about various food groups were not made. Such recommendations are made in Table 36. This table illustrates the plan that the I propose for weight reduction and cardiovascular health combined. The key to the plan is that it is not merely a diet but an adjustment of the calorie intake of the diet that will make the dietary plan effective at weight control.

·    A special health role exists for soy, essential fatty acids and soluble fiber (beta glucan fractions of soluble fiber).

·    Low saturated fat, normal protein intake of vegetable preference, low simple sugars, high complex carbohydrate, low salt and cholesterol conscious. Varying foods preferred.

·    Calorie intake reduction is the key to weight loss. Calorie intakes of less than 1500 calories per day require supervision of a healthcare professional.

·    Avoid dieting pills or dietary supplements with false claims.

·    Educate yourself in calorie contents and nutritional values of foods. Read labels on food.

·    Train yourself to eat properly, e.g. only when hungry, chew well, make a meal on occasion.

·    Decrease intake of: animal foods, fried foods, and especially beef, cheese, butter and margarine. Watch for more 'unhealthy' fruits, e.g. avocado, coconut and nuts high in saturated fat. Avoid alcohol, food colorants, additives or sugar.

·    Increase intake of: vegetables, fish, grains and low fat, non-salted, fresh nuts. The author believes that most approved artificial sweeteners are safe.

- Supplement Western Diets with fiber (>25 gm/day), use beta glucan fractions of soluble fiber, soy protein (25 gm/day), omega 3 and omega 6 oils in varying ways described in this book.

**Table 36:** Some Specific "Dietary Recommendations", without succumbing to the need for menus.

## THE COMBAT SYNDROME X DIET

In this chapter, I have not committed to a single dietary recommendation for reasons that I trust have become obvious. Diets must be made to fit to an individuals' needs. However, we can start to define dietary principles and recommendations for macronutrient intakes in terms of calories and ratios of inclusion (the amount and type of fat, carbohydrates and protein in the diet) to combat Syndrome X. The general principles that are applied in a diet to combat Syndrome X involve:

- A reduction of carbohydrate intake in the form of simple sugars. About 40-50% of the diet can come from carbohydrates preferably of the complex type.

- Eat foods with a low glycemic index. Foods that cause high swings in blood glucose and promote insulin secretion make syndrome X worse. Substitute complex carbohydrates and fiber.

- Intakes of "healthy types of fats" can be more liberal than proposed in nationally acclaimed diets e.g. USDA Food Pyramid or American Heart Association. Dr. Reaven has proposed that an effective diet to combat Syndrome X may derive 40% of its calories from fat, but he stresses healthy fat.

- Only 10-15% of the diet needs to come from protein. Excessive protein intake especially of meat or dairy origin is linked to many chronic degenerative diseases and components of protein (certain amino acids) can cause insulin release.

I reiterate my belief that all fixed dietary recommendations possess disadvantages or limitations and I stress the need to obtain expert nutritional advice to tailor a diet to an individuals' needs. The limitations of some diets are illustrated by comparisons of popular diets that have been proposed, even including some recently recommended diets to combat Syndrome X (Table 37).

| Macronutrient Popular diets | Components | Comments |
| --- | --- | --- |
| The Zone Diet | 30% protein, 30% fat and 40% carbohydrate | A step in the right direction for Syndrome X. Too high in protein which can release insulin. |
| The Atkins Diet | 25% protein 55% fat or more and less than 20% carbohydrate | The low carbohydrate (simple sugar) aspect of this diet is its only merit. |
| The American Heart Association Diet | 15% protein, < 30%fat, up to 60% carbohydrate | Questioned on carbohydrate content |
| The Syndrome X-Diet (Reaven Diet) , | 5% protein, 40%fat, 45% carbohydrate | Moves towards more healthy fat, diet expanded by Mr. Jack Challem and colleagues |
| American Dietetic Association | No fixed calories or ratios, uses expert advice and exchange lists | Expert advice is the advantage now that dieticians recognize the issue of insulin resistance, this could be optimal |

| American Diabetes Association | Same as American Dietetic Association | Expert advice is the advantage, tailored for the diabetic |
|---|---|---|

**Table 37: Components and comments about popular diets. The "New** Age" of dietary advice is becoming "mainstream", at last !

I admit that there is no consensus on the ideal diet for lowering cholesterol, or impacting Syndrome X. This lack of consensus should not provoke arguments, but it should finally help the "penny drop" with the knowledge that there is no single, universally beneficial diet plan. All diets are of limited value without a complete program of treatment.

The work of Dr. G. Reaven on the Syndrome X diet questions the alleged widespread benefits of the American Heart Association (AHA) Diet and its modification as the Ornish Program. However, there is some outcome research to support the benefits of the AHA diet and the Ornish Program, but how much of this benefit is due to the diet or other factors is not entirely clear.

Out of this lack of consensus certain issues become clear but the real issue is that diets must be matched to individuals' needs – "horses for courses." I propose the following issues to be considered:

1) Cutting back on dietary saturated fats and cholesterol (the foundation of the AHA diet) is beneficial. This clear fact disqualifies the Atkins Diet from being heart healthy, but Dr. Atkins has in recent times stressed the value of healthy fats of the omega 3 series. The AHA will not "come clean" on the negative consequences of refined carbohydrates.

2) Excessive protein intake does not, itself, cause weight loss, it is associated with chronic disease (e.g. osteoporosis) and it often comes along with fat. These issues tend to make the Zone Diet an unrealistic option. Furthermore, proteins can be broken down to amino acids that will promote insulin secretion. Excessive animal protein is best avoided in Syndrome X, but the same may not be true of vegetable protein, e.g. soy protein,

which may have favorable effects on insulin and glucagon release by virtue of its lower content of sulfur containing amino acids.

3) The type of fat in the diet is much more important than previously recognized. Mono and polyunsaturated fats (oils) that are not adulterated (hydrogenated to form trans fatty acids) are generally healthy. However, the omega 6 to omega 3 unsaturated fatty acid balance is very important (see Section 8, Essential Fatty Acids in Natural Options for Syndrome X).

4) Diets to curb insulin resistance must limit simple sugars, saturated fats and salt, but may contain more liberal amounts of "healthy fat," with careful concern for their calorie content to avoid weight gain. Protein metabolism in the presence of glucose intolerance is often disturbed and excessive protein intake may be undesirable.

5) The "glycemic index" of food is an important principle which measures the ability of any given food to shoot up levels of blood glucose and insulin, (see Section 7, The Secret of Soluble Fiber).

6) Selected dietary supplements and functional foods are of value in the "first line attack" against the components of Syndrome X e.g. soluble fiber, beta glucan fractions of soluble oat fiber, soy protein, omega 3 fatty acids (see Sections 7 and 8). This proposal somewhat confronts conservative opinions of some nutritionists and healthcare givers. Syndrome X Nutritional Factors.

Overall, the diet to combat Syndrome X does not exist as a stand alone intervention. Leading healthcare organizations and many researchers stress programs with lifestyle change and perhaps other natural options.

## What One Can Do

Table 38 gives specific and simple instructions on what individual can do to start their combat against Syndrome X.

 

– Educate yourself in nutrition
– Answer the following:         Am I Fat?
                                        Do I have Syndrome X?

– How fat ? and How much at risk may I be? (Ask a healthcare giver)

· What are my dietary objectives, goals and what is my timetable? (You can ask a healthcare giver)

· Have I eliminated other cardiovascular risk factors? (e.g. smoking, excessive stress)

· Can I decide on the lifestyle change and modify my behavior accordingly? (It's make your mind up time)

· Do I know enough about food facts and fallacies? (You can ask a healthcare giver)

· Create your plan.

· Go to work on the plan.

· What Foods? (See recommendations on the Combat Syndrome X diet)

· Are extracts soluble fiber or of soluble fiber, essential fatty acids (omega 3) and soy healthful? (Ask a healthcare giver who took the time to find out the answer)

**Table 38:** Some key steps in the proposed "Combat Syndrome X Diet Plan".

## CHAPTER SUMMARY

Obesity is challenging the health of Western society. The last thing we need in this millennium is to keep the confusion going about the "ideal" diet. Such a diet does not exist. Public education on nutrition is imperative if we are to control our weight. This may help people tailor their diet to their specific needs. The emerging importance of Syndrome X has changed our view of macronutrient intake with a recognition of the benefits of reducing simple sugar and salt intake whilst watching the "quality" of fat intake in the diet. The "fad nature" and fallacies of some popular diets must be recognized.

# SECTION 6

# LIFESTYLE TO COMBAT SYNDROME X

## The Lifestyle Concept

Physical and mental well-being are regarded as the greatest treasures of life, but many people seem reluctant to take control of sociobehavioral factors that promote ill health. These factors are essentially lifestyle issues. Lifestyle has a direct influence on health. This situation is easily overlooked because the effects of adverse or poor lifestyle on an individual are not often immediate. In other words, positive action to change adverse lifestyle for the better does not often produce rapid results. Furthermore, many forms of adverse lifestyle are pleasurable. An individual can exert complete control over his or her lifestyle, but exerting this control is often difficult. Adverse lifestyle is the commonest cause of preventable disease. Therefore, it is of utmost importance that harmful lifestyle be clearly identified and interventions to enact positive lifestyle should occur early with simple and effective corrective actions (Skinner HA, Holt S, Journal of the Royal College of General Practitioners, 33, 787-91, 1983).

Lifestyle is a general concept that encompasses psychological, physical and social functioning. Each person's lifestyle is different and several domains exist which are illustrated in Table 39. All lifestyle domains constitute the global concept of lifestyle and their assessment has a bearing on physical and mental health, e.g., substance abuse, drug abuse, nutrition, exercise, etc. These domains

are interrelated and in many cases interdependent. My colleagues
and I have researched lifestyle interventions with a particular focus
on alcohol problems, but whatever the adverse lifestyle issues the
principles of identification and intervention are portable. It is recognized that the interplay of cardiovascular risk factors in
Syndrome X operates through an interplay of many components of
an unhealthy lifestyle.

Many attempts have been made to measure or check lifestyle
in the population, but one efficient method involves the comparison of an individual's components of lifestyle with those of the general population. This measurement technique has the advantage of
showing us that there are "degrees" of poor lifestyle. This process
of comparison should not be perceived as an "all or nothing" phenomenon. Clearly, the more areas of an individual's lifestyle that
are under the influence of positive action, the better off an individual will be or feel! There are some problems in defining adverse
lifestyle accurately and what is perceived by some as "normal"
lifestyle may not be healthy. For example, a safe level of alcohol
consumption defies accurate definition and many individuals see
daily fast food intake as "normal nutrition".

| | |
|---|---|
| 1. Consumption | 4. Nutrition/Eating |
| 2. Psychological Well-Being | 5. Sexual Activity |
| 3. Substance Abuse | 6. Physical Activity/Exercise |

**Table 39:** The Principle Lifestyle Domains

## Assessing One's Lifestyle: Self–Watching

The assessment of adverse lifestyle such as smoking or excessive drinking is applied variably in a medical clinic by a doctor or
a nurse (Skinner HA, Holt S, Sheu WJ and Israel Y, British Medical
journal, 292, 1703-8, 1986). The most efficient method of lifestyle
assessment is probably self-identification of a problem followed by
self-intervention, a process that requires self-education in health
matters. "Behavioral Assessment Research" has shown that stan-
dardized questions with feedback are known to be the preferred
way of measuring the magnitude of a lifestyle problem. Modern
technology has helped us in lifestyle assessment. In fact, it is possi-

ble to have questions written into a computer software program where the computer interrogates the patient about lifestyle.

The computer is capable of monotonous questioning about lifestyle in a precise manner.  My colleagues and I have developed a computer-assisted lifestyle testing program that has been shown to be useful in assessing lifestyle in clinic patients.  Most patients rated the experience as acceptable and the results of a study suggested that a patient may tell more to a computer than to a doctor! The use of the computer-assisted testing of lifestyle resulted in prompting patients to discuss concerns with their doctors that they may otherwise have failed to bring up in a routine clinic visit (Holt S, Guram M, Smith MA and Skinner HA, Digestive Diseases and Sciences, 37, 7, 993-996, 1992).

## THE 10 LIFESTYLE COMMANDMENTS

An enormous amount of epidemiological (population studies)research has linked a wide variety of behaviors, addictions or compulsions with the causation of chronic degenerative disease. These realizations have underscored the importance of advances in experimental and clinical psychology that permit a process of behavioral change. This change of behavior is based on practical, "common-sense" advice and help.   Any attempts to change ingrained habits requires great commitment and motivation. However, it is now recognized that a simple commitment is not enough, clear plans of action are required to enact corrections of adverse lifestyle.  In other words, being told what to do is one thing, but being told how to do it is another. The "how to" is missing in many popular books on lifestyle change.

I have prepared a list of lifestyle "commandments" which were developed from a consideration of the many examples of adverse lifestyles that are known to be harmful to health.  At first sight these lifestyle commandments may be perceived to be general recommendations for health.  The well kept secret is that general health recommendations cross over completely to cardiovascular wellness and the combat against Syndrome X.  The 10 lifestyle commandments are summarized in Table 40. These commandments are not proposed with any religious connotation, though each piece of advice occurs in one form or another in the bible.

1.      Control your drinking of alcohol or abstain if you have recognized a problem.
2.      Avoid substance abuse, e.g., excesses of caffeine-containing beverages, unnecessary use of dietary supplements, over-the-counter or prescription medications, etc.
3.      Stop smoking.
4.      Exercise regularly and consistently.
5.      Be in touch with your moods and levels of "stress". Simplify your life if you can.
6.      Eat because you are hungry and eat only to satisfy your appetite.
7.      Eat a healthy balanced diet high in fiber, low in sodium, cholesterol and saturated fat.
8.      Subject yourself to a periodic health examination, e.g., an annual physical.
9.      Practice monogamy or safe sex.
10.     Never "do" drugs.

**Table 40:** The 10 Lifestyle Commandments

## SELF–IDENTIFICATION AND SELF–INTERVENTION

Several psychologists have written excellent accounts of the art of self-watching and self-help. Authors, philosophers and psychologists refer consistently to the issues of "self-knowledge" which can create "inner values" that will change behavior. These are pivotal issues in starting to combat adverse lifestyles that operate within the domains of Syndrome X and other causes of ill health.

Behavioral scientists have wrestled with their understanding of the persistence of adverse lifestyle in the face of the individual's knowledge that the consequences of the unhealthy behavior can be catastrophic. Alcohol abusers may lose their jobs and family and smokers may often get heart disease and lung cancer. Smokers "bond" whilst they "hang" out in areas displaced from "no smoking" zones, but they are acutely aware of their "outcast status". However, the power of the addiction overcomes their social discomfort. The answer to this enigma of complacency to persist with adverse lifestyle may lie in an understanding of the temporal (timing) relationship between the poor habit and the reward it gives.

Understanding the processes of reinforcement of adverse lifestyle can assist an individual in his or her own intervention for better health. Immediate pleasure from an adverse lifestyle, such as smoking, may far outweigh any considerations of harm in the long-term. Thus, short-term gratification is a powerful reinforcer of adverse lifestyle. A common example of this circumstance is eating fast (junk) food. Eating fast food (or junk food) today leads to obesity and ill health that is not apparent tomorrow. The negative health consequences of excessive simple sugar and saturated fat in the diet is apparent only over a period of months or years. It is easy to pile "on the beef", but hard to lose it!

## ALCOHOL, CAFFEINE AND HEART DISEASE

There are many medical reasons to avoid excessive drinking of alcohol in the presence of heart disease or in the presence of risk factors for cardiovascular disorders. Excessive drinking is strongly correlated with excessive smoking and alcohol is directly toxic to cardiac muscle. Elegant clinical experiments show that acute alcohol intake can have profound effects on cardiovascular responses by dilating blood vessels and depressing myocardial (heart muscle) performance. On occasion, alcohol can trigger abnormal heart rhythm and the effects of alcohol on the central nervous system can unleash behavioral activity that places a susceptible individual at acute risk of a heart attack or bodily injury.

Much has been made of the potential beneficial effects of alcohol on cardiac function and blood lipids. Reports that red wine contain beneficial antioxidants (OPC's, see Section 8) with cardiovascular benefit is not an excuse to gulp a bottle of wine with each meal. Studies, including those of my colleagues and I, have shown that modest alcohol intake raises HDL, but it does not normalize blood lipids and, therefore, the evidence for benefit is somewhat arguable. However, I do not reject drinking at social levels - one or two drinks, no more than three times a week – a best guess at "safe drinking" (Holt S, Skinner HA and Israel Y, Canadian Medical Association Journal 124, 10, 1279-94, 1981).

There are no merits associated with coffee or cola drinking for the person at risk of cardiovascular disease. One alarming study undertaken in Norway indicated that coffee consumption is a predictor of coronary death and it operates at a level more than can be explained by its known effects on raising blood cholesterol or blood pressure. Caffeine containing beverages may whip up the "fright and flight" reaction in the body and it stresses the adrenal glands. Hormones released from the adrenal glands (catectolamines and cortisol) tend to raise blood sugar. This "rush" may be pleasant, but it is not regarded as healthy, especially in the presence of insulin resistance. Unfortunately, decaffeinated coffee does not clearly afford protection. The jury remains out on the caffeine content of coffee or cola and cardiovascular risk. However, caffeine, in coffee or cola, is to be avoided in the individual with established heart disease because it can alter heart rate and rhythm, as well as increase platelet reactivity (platelet stickiness is associated with blood clotting). One may recall that Syndrome X is associated with an increased tendency to blood clotting.

## Smoker's Heart Attack

Smoking is associated with an increased prevalence of coronary artery disease, but it emerges as a very significant risk factor in the precipitation of acute heart attack (myocardial infarction). It has been argued inappropriately by some individuals that smoking cessation in later life is not associated with much benefit. Recent studies have shown this not to be the case. Clinical studies show that people who quite smoking in adult life have a measurable reduction in the risk of coronary artery disease after about two years of smoking cessation. Furthermore, quitting smoking in individuals who are in mid-life results in an overall improvement in life expectancy of at least two years.

There is much benefit to be obtained by stopping smoking in Syndrome X, Y and Z..., but medical interventions for smoking cessation are notoriously unsuccessful. There have been questions about the cost-effectiveness of medical treatment for smoking cessation because many treatments are effective only in somewhere between one in twenty and one in five individuals. However, the benefits that accrue from the discontinuation of cigarette smoking are so significant that medical interventions for smoking cessation are best perceived as cost-effective, despite their low success rate.

## SUBSTANCE ABUSE

Is it legal or illegal? Legalities and morals may matter less than slow death or serious impairment of day-to-day life that occurs with illicit drug use or misuse of prescription or over the counter drugs (or dietary supplements !). Everyone has the potential to become addicted to certain drugs. Any kind of addiction is self-defeating and dangerous to well-being and happiness. Drug addiction or misuse are among the biggest problems facing humankind and it is responsible for much privation, premature death and social misery. The role of drug use in Syndrome X requires much further study, but one could predict that many drugs will make the components of Syndrome X worse.

The term "addiction" has been superseded in many fields of medicine by the kinder term "dependence". Addiction is a better term for most purposes because it reinforces the recognition that something nefarious has gained a strong, habitual and enduring hold - the hold is <u>STRONG</u>, it is a <u>HABIT</u> and it is <u>ENDURING</u>. Counter-activity must, therefore, be as strong as the habit. A commitment to stop substance abuse needs to be applied repeatedly, without relent, if an individual is to be successful in breaking the "addiction". I mention substance abuse because I believe it to be an underestimated risk factor for cardiovascular disease within the "bouquet of barbed wire".

## EXERCISE

Exercise can make important contributions to all aspects physical and mental well-being. Before commencing an exercise program, it is important that the individual checks with his or her physician. A physician will be able to give some advice about the type and amount of exercise that is ideal. There are some misconceptions about the role of exercise in lifestyle. An individual may set an expectation that is too great and it is known that an individual's ability to undertake an exercise depends on his or her physical condition, age and general health. Unlike sportsmen or women who need to train very arduously, most individuals should not push exercise to the limits.

Exercise has a very beneficial direct effect on the heart, lungs, muscles, joints and bones. Exercise is a very important adjunct to diet in a weight loss program because calories are expended and fat accumulation will not tend to occur or may diminish. Exercise is an important aid to rehabilitation following any illness. If exercise is sustained for at least 15 minutes, it results in improvements in cardiovascular and respiratory function of the body. In addition, exercise helps lower blood sugar and prevent diabetes mellitus – and Syndrome X. Routine daily exercise or workouts have a preventative benefit in terms of respiratory and circulatory diseases. Exercise increases circulation and improves muscle tone and strength. It is possible to benefit from exercise in many different forms, including walking, housework, jogging, biking, swimming or doing a series of stretching exercises.

Regular exercise, even if it is not strenuous, will help burn calories and plays an important adjunctive role in dieting and the management of obesity. Thus, exercise is a great helper in the combat against Syndrome X. There is a common misconception that a workout has to be strenuous in order to burn calories, but this is not necessarily the case, especially for the reformed "couch potato". It is quite useful to keep a daily log of exercise activity and certain goals can be set to achieve over a period of time. A daily activity-diary should contain information on the date, time at which exercise occurs, description of the exercise or activity, a note of the number of times that exercise occurs and a comment as to whether or not the exercise was easy or difficult. It is possible to calculate the number of calories that are burned with different forms of exercise from several different types of activity chart.

## THE ARDENT EXERCISE FAN

Facilities for aerobic exercise have sprung up all over the place in recent years. The duplication of gymnasium-type facilities is a good trend, but some evidence exists that certain methods used in aerobic exercise routines and attempts to enhance peak physical performance may not be healthy. Some of the nutritional advice given to the sports enthusiast requires a careful reappraisal and I believe that some young athletes may be trading future health for body contours.

The dangers and putative advantages of some nutritional

techniques to improve muscle bulk (mass) are not well defined. Excessive protein loading may have marginal benefits to enhance lean body mass, but it is not known to be healthy. I believe that much more attention must be placed on nutritional principals to support cardiovascular health and combat Syndrome X in the "exercising" enthusiast.

Dangerous practices in the ardent exercisers include the taking of anabolic steroids or hormone containing dietary supplements, the use of energizers to improve performance (e.g. Ephedra or Ma Huang, Guarana and Tribulus terrestris) and fad diets that ignore "heart-healthy" principles. The gymnasium should not become a breeding ground for Syndrome X, Y and Z... that is increasingly affecting our Generation Y. Some nutritional advice given in "fitness magazines" is more than a "brick short of a load" !

## PSYCHOLOGICAL WELL-BEING

The mind controls the body. In fact, the mind can make the body do almost anything. Psychological well-being for most people implies a state of happiness and moderate contentment. Much of the time, however, life is not perfect. It is normal to perceive life as experiencing some ups and downs. The negative effect of anxiety, stress and depression has become clear. The idea of the "broken heart" as a consequence of emotional or psychological problems transmits into a break in a cardiac health. There are many types of stressful life events (e.g. divorce, job loss etc.) which can have a cumulative effect on health and these issues figure in the precipitation and progression of Syndrome X, in a poorly defined manner. Mind-body medicine (psycho-neuroimmunoendocrinology) is an extremely important component of healthcare that is just dawning on many medical practitioners.

## BEHAVIOR THAT WILL GET YOU IN THE END

In order to change thoughts and, therefore, feelings, an individual may have to change his or her habits or exposure to environmental influences, in a radical manner. There are some simple facts about living a happy life with contentment. Tips on happiness are an important component of cardiovascular wellness. An individual does well to adopt the no complaining stance. It is easy to complain. Complaints are much easier than positive attitudes in the face of disappointment. If one is not happy, one cannot be healthy.

## TYPE A BEHAVIOR AND CARDIOVASCULAR DISEASE

Dr. Friedman and Dr. Rosenman (1974) paved the way to an understanding of the importance of Type A behavior in the causation of coronary heart disease. These doctors were so convinced that cardiovascular disease had its roots in aggressive, impatient temperaments, that they proposed the following in the preface of their classic book titled, "Type A Behavior and Your Heart". Friedman and Rosenman (1974) state "In the absence of Type A Behavior Pattern, coronary heart disease almost never occurs before seventy years of age, regardless of the fatty foods eaten, the cigarettes smoked, or the lack of exercise. But when this behavior pattern is present, coronary heart disease can easily erupt in one's thirties or forties." These statements are sweeping and partially correct. However, Type A behavior and Syndrome X are a particularly destructive combination that act against heart health.

The main features of Type A behavior are summarized in Table 41. A study of this table highlights the complexity of Type A behavior which has been termed an "action-emotion complex". An important component of the behavior pattern is that minor challenges in the environment may provoke explosive reactions in the Type A personality.

| Feature | Comment |
|---|---|
| Time urgency | This is regarded as the key aspect of Type A behavior. Not enough seconds in a minute! |
| Accentuation of words in speaking | Typically hurries to finish a sentence |
| Rapid eating, walking and movement | Easy to spot in the Type A |

| | |
|---|---|
| Overt impatience | Want people to get on with what they are saying or doing |
| Doing or thinking more than one thing at once | The individual contaminates leisure time with thoughts of work or problems. |
| Conversation focusing | The individual brings the theme of a conversation to egocentric topics |
| Inappropriate guilt | Cannot rest without discomfort |
| Cannot smell the "roses" | The individual must have things here and now |
| Creating tight schedules | More and more appointments in less time. |
| The face that makes people feel like punching it! | The Type A person is challenging and does not engender sympathy for his or her own affliction |
| Tics and Gestures | Finger pointing, table thumping and jaw protrusion are examples of the innate aggression |
| Belief that speed gives an edge | The Type A person has to move quicker than anyone |
| Measuring others deeds | The Type A person may apply numbers to activities, or actions thoughts or deeds |
| Type A plus Type A | The Type A is rapidly engaged by his fellow Type A. This causes "sparks" |

**Table 41: Main features of Type A behavior that are modified from** Friedman and Rosenman (1974). The comments provide examples of the behavior.

A study of the opposite type of behavior to Type A behavior may be a good way of identifying and correcting adverse behavioral traits. The opposite type of behavior has been termed Type B. It has been recognized that Type B personality is much less likely to get coronary heat disease than the Type A individual, even in the face of similar cardiovascular risk factors.

The Type B person is not necessarily outwardly docile. Indeed, this person may have greater ambition than the Type A individual, but he or she is not obsessed with the "here and now" and does not engage in the activity of doing ever-increasing numbers of things in ever-decreasing amounts of time. Switching from Type A to Type B behavior is the ideal solution, but taking the edge off the Type A tendency is probably all that is required. The desirable components of the Type B personality are summarized in Table 42 . Which type are you? - bearing in mind that 10-20% of the population have an intricate mixture of Type A and Type B tendencies and, like Syndrome X, neither pattern may breed true entirely.

- The Type B trait is free of Type A habits and activities
- No sense of time urgency
- Does not experience free floating hostility
- Does not need to keep discussing victories or topics of self-interest
- No need to portray themselves as superior
- Relaxes without guilt
- Works efficiently but steadily
- Not necessarily docile or "brain dead"

**Table 42:** The Type B behavior pattern, as modified from Freidman and Rosenman (1974).

## THE MIND MINDS THE HEART

Dr. Deepak Chopra, M.D., is commended with his popularization of Ayurvedic medicine which stresses the importance of emotional factors, thought and awareness in general health. In his classic book titled, "Ageless Body, Timeless Mind…", Dr. Chopra teaches much about "awareness" as a secret to longevity. I subscribe more to the Dalai Lama's proposals of inner values that emanate from enlightenment. The assertion of mind-control over body processes (structures and functions) is believed to exert a holistic and positive influence on health. The notion that the mind-body system reacts with generalization to even a simple stimulus has become increasingly accepted. A good example of a single stimulus with general health benefit is exercise. Lack of exercise or even simple mobility can have a devastating effect on the body. Recent scientific studies show us that exercise is a key antidote to Syndrome X. The mature individual that sits in a chair with no stimuli will develop a decreasing awareness and deterioration of physical health. This knowledge supports the perception of Syndrome X as a form of X-Degeneration where lack of exercise is a cause.

Physical activity is used as an example of one simple stimulus since the outcome sedentary habits are readily identifiable. Of equal, if not more importance, could be lack of psychological well-being itself due to limited social interaction, or other factors. The circumstances become even more complex when lack of psychological well-being is perceived as endogenous (from within). The principal antidote to depression is activity. Mind-body interactions form an intricate web inside the "bouquet of barbed wire" and they are operative in the progression of Syndrome X. Inactivity, be it emotional or physical, will lead to reductions in mental or physical well-being. Above all, the mind is the minder of the body.

## SPIRITUAL CONNECTION

The role of love and prayer in healing and wellness is a developing science. According to Dr. Larry Dossey, "Love makes it possible for the mind to transcend the limitations of the body." Dr. Dossey is the author of the book titled, "The Power of Prayer and the Practice of Medicine" (1993) and he was the Chairman of the National Institutes of Health Office Panel on Mind-Body Interventions. Dr. Dossey believes in the power of love to create health. He draws attention to the finding that in a study of 10,000 males with cardiac disease there was a 50 percent observed reduction in the frequency of anginal chest pain in men who recognized their spouses as loving and supportive. Prayer may conjure up the notion that this intervention is only available to the individual with religious inclination. The involvement of religion reinforces belief in prayer and must make it more effective, but belief systems of different religious connotations are all valuable. Atheists must be clever people or perhaps misguided people?

## LOVE, SEX, AND THE HEART

While we appear to live in a society that seems overly preoccupied with sex, many people in the United States have grown up in a sexually repressive atmosphere. Because of this somewhat puritanical climate, many men and women do not easily discuss sexual matters. But for those fortunate enough to have a loving relationship with a life partner, the warmth of love and sex can play a powerful – and natural – role in healing. Men and women should be encouraged to explore their sexual attitudes and take advantage of new information about maintaining and enhancing sexual health. Sexual health is linked to general health

Dr. Dean Ornish MD, the famous cardiologist, has explored the role of love and emotional intimacy in his book "Love and Survival". Loving relationships with a partner, children, parents, friends, and associates are among the best stress management tools. "Love and Survival" explores many concepts, including techniques to improve communication and listening skills and other ways to strengthen intimate connections. There is no question that loneliness, isolation, and lack of intimacy with others contributes to heart disease. Developing and enriching relationships with others is at least as important as exercise routines.

Unfortunately, the consequences of Syndrome X often damage sexual health. Glucose intolerance and diabetes mellitus are a common cause of vascular disorders that cause erectile dysfunction. Cardiovascular health is mandatory for normal sexual function. Furthermore, Syndrome X causes infertility in females and it is associated with polycystic ovary syndrome (PCOS, see Section 1). Thus, sexual health is interwoven with Syndrome X and an effective combat against Syndrome X, Y and Z... will improve sexual well-being and vice versa.

## Remember the Bouquet of Barbed Wire

Obesity, high blood cholesterol and, surprising to some, malnutrition go hand in hand. The interesting outcome that emerges from the effective reversal of cardiovascular risk factors is that their global reduction results in a beneficial results for general health. However, global reductions occur in complex interdependent manners. For example, exercise burns calories and assists in weight reduction, stopping smoking improves exercise tolerance, and reduction of caloric intake causes weight loss and lowers cholesterol. One can now re-examine the value of the overall concept of Syndrome X, where it is known that complex interdependent risks exist in a way that is amenable to correction by many positive lifestyle factors. .

All of this sounds simple but several traps exist when lifestyle changes are made. Quitting smoking often leads to weight gain. Exercise may increase appetite and some diets that are designed for weight loss result in rebound weight gain. Smoking with excessive coffee consumption is a popular, quite pleasurable, but very unhealthy way to lose weight. I believe that the overall answer to Syndrome X and other cardiovascular risk factors rests primarily in a carefully planned combination of a nutritional and lifestyle program. Good nutrition impacts Syndrome X and assists in the fight against flab, the smoothing of temperament, the struggle with substance abuse and the promotion of a general feeling of well-being. There is no doubt that optimal nutrition is necessary for optimum health.

## Behavior Modification Guidelines for Weight Control

In Section 5, we discussed "Obesity and the Slim Chance" with recommendations that moved "back to basics". I stress that successful weight control can only occur by modifications of day to day habits, especially eating behavior. Many individuals develop strong eating habits that work against efforts to control calorie intake and promote exercise. Several specific suggestions can be reiterated on behavior modification as part of a weight control plan:

- Recognize calorie contents of various foods and establish a target for calorie intake. It is necessary to review on a regular basis whether or not calorie intake goals have been met.
- Choose low calorie, high glycemic index foods and if snacking is planned then healthy reduced caloric snacks must be used.
- Avoid "temptations" or external influences that precipitate eating. Plan what you want to eat rather than selecting from set menus and prepare only as much food as meets the calorie goals that have been set.
- Think about calories not about food and treat yourself for meeting the calorie intake. Do not use food as a reward.
- Heighten your awareness of body feelings that make you eat. Do not eat past hunger signals. Pause during a meal and ask yourself if your appetite is satisfied.
- Use your imagination creatively. Imagine that you feel lousy after overeating – remember the feeling. Look in a mirror when you want to binge or imagine that you have just eaten.
- Do not take two steps forward and three back. Accept occasional failures and never permit them to be an excuse to give up.
- Problem solve with a greater awareness of your ability to reason. Do not succumb to victimizing statements about weight.
- Every failure must be a lesson learned. Educate yourself about nutrition and lifestyle or review what you know.

## Chapter Summary

Changing lifestyle is an important component in the combat against Syndrome X. The complacency about the cardinal features of Syndrome X (obesity, insulin resistance, hypertension and high blood cholesterol) is transcended by even greater complacency about poor lifestyle habits. Preventing disease, especially those diseases linked to Syndrome X, Y and Z…, is not possible without fundamental movements toward positive lifestyle choices. Failure to address the sociobehavioral issues that cause disease is responsible for the stubbornly high occurrence of cardiovascular disease and Syndrome X.

# SECTION 7:

# THE SECRET
# OF SOLUBLE FIBER

## THE FIBER HYPOTHESIS

Several scientists have proposed that a deficiency of plant fiber in the diet may predispose individuals to many of the chronic degenerative diseases that afflict Western society. The fiber hypothesis, as first proposed, was dependent for its support on scientific information derived from population studies and medical practice experiences. Drawing conclusions from the occurrence of certain disease profiles in Western culture (fiber deficient), compared with those in more primitive cultures (fiber abundant), assisted in supporting and clarifying the modern "fiber hypothesis". This "modern hypothesis" was proposed principally by Dr. Dennis P. Burkitt MD, but it is a renaissance in thought from earlier reports of the health benefits of fiber.

On average, a vegetarian consumes more than twice the amount of fiber as an individual who consumes a recommended healthy Western diet (greater than 40 g/day versus much less than 20 g/day). In more traditional cultures, such as those of African natives, the daily dietary fiber intake ranges from 50 to 150 g/day, especially when maize is the dietary staple. When fiber is mentioned, the average person thinks mainly about digestive health. It is interesting to note that the stool weight of many Westerners may be 100 g/day or less, whereas the African native eating maize diets may pass up to 1 kg or more of stool per day. However, the health benefits

of fiber consumption in the diet go far beyond any benefits on
dumping stool or gastrointestinal function.

Comparisons of the diets of white and black South Africans
have shown that as urbanization of the black person occurs, the diet
changes to increase the amount and proportion of fat and protein
intake. In addition, the diet becomes enhanced in refined carbohydrate (simple sugar) intake, and the total dietary fiber intake falls
dramatically. Coincidental with these dietary changes, the urban
black develops a disease profile similar to that of the urban white.
Disorders, such as colon cancer, bowel problems, and heart disease,
tend to increase in incidence as dietary fiber intake is reduced. A key
recent and predictable finding is that Syndrome X is appearing
increasingly in black South African people (and white South
Africans).

Dietary fiber in a variety of forms has been shown to reduce
blood cholesterol, and it may play a major role in the prevention
of colon cancer, gallstones, inflammatory bowel disease, diverticular disease, diabetes mellitus, varicose veins, and functional gastrointestinal disease (spastic colon, irritable bowel syndrome). Fiber
has an established therapeutic role in the treatment of diverticular
disease, colitis, constipation, and functional bowel disease. It is beg-
ging to be recognized as a major antidote to Syndrome X, when
administered as mixtures of soluble fiber or fractions of bioactive
soluble fiber (beta glucans).

## INCREASING DIETARY FIBER INTAKE

There are several ways to increase fiber in the diet. First, an
individual may elect to seek dietary components that are rich in
insoluble and soluble fibers. This is a difficult goal for the average
person and it often involves moving somewhat towards a vegetarian diet. Because of the impracticalities of deriving fiber from natural food sources, many individuals have adopted a habit of
predictable fiber intake in the form of dietary supplements.
Unprocessed types of bran are desirable for their health benefit,
but they are unpalatable. Several types of fiber in the diet can be
isolated for use in dietary supplements and their properties are
shown in Table 43.

| Preparation | Description | Contact with water |
| --- | --- | --- |
| Bran fiber | Fibrous outer layer of cereal grains, usually wheat | Poorly soluble with water holding dependent on particle size. |
| Plantago Species (Ispaghula) P. ovata P. pysllium P. indica | Small dried ripe seeds; cellulose-containing walls of endosperm and mucilage-containing epidermis | Colorless transparent mucilage forms around insoluble seed. A sticky, dense concoction. |
| Ispaghula Husk | Epidermis and collapsed adjacent layer of Plantago species | Swells rapidly to form a stiff mucilage |
| Sterculia Gum | Gum obtained from Sterculia species | Forms a homogeneous, adhesive gelatinous mass |
| Methylcellulose | Methyl ether of cellulose | Slowly soluble, giving a viscous, colloidal solution |
| Soluble oat fibers (extracts) | Glucocolloids containing beta glucans | These modern extracts of soluble fiber form a bulky drink with a pleasant mouth feel (like fat). |

(continued)

| Mixed soluble and insoluble | Oat fiber (Oligofiber™) | Ideal bowel regulators, with bulk advantage of insoluble and soluble fiber action |

**Table 43: Fiber Supplement Ingredients. A form of bioactive fiber that** has versatile and potent benefits in Syndrome X is soluble oat fiber extract (glucocolloids composed of beta glucans). Whilst many commercial fiber supplements contain healthy fiber ingredients, some of those sold as "pharmaceuticals" contain artificial additives and coloring which may not be healthy. Readers are asked to read labels on products.

## FIBER IS RESISTANT TO DIGESTION

The forms of fiber that are of major interest in the potential promotion of cardiovascular health are the soluble types of fiber found in oats (especially beta glucan fractions)and bean fiber, eg guar gum. Oat derived fiber shares many of the physical properties of other plant-derived fibers, which are characterized by their water-holding ability and their resistance to digestion. The resistance of fiber to digestion causes bulking of the stool. Individuals who consume water-holding (hydrophilic) indigestible fiber have more bulky stool and the weight of stool passed in a 24-hour period is substantially increased by the addition of fiber to the diet.

Dietary fiber is generally derived from the supporting structures of vegetation. These supporting structures are often found in the coverings of vegetables and are abundant in the stems and leaves of plants. Overall, fiber is composed of plant polysaccharides (complex sugars) and lignins that are not amenable to easy degradation by digestive enzymes of the human gastrointestinal tract. However, fiber can be degraded by bacteria (fermented), which are abundant in the large intestine (colon) of humans. Although the bacterial decomposition of fiber (fermentation) in the colon may produce minor gas and bloating of the abdomen, it also produces important health-giving short chain fatty acids (SCFA). These SCFA are absorbed into the body from the colon and they are responsible for several effects of soluble fiber on body chemistry. They account for part of the "intrinsic metabolic effects" of fiber (IMEF). These IMEF are effects on body functions that occur independent of the physical properties of fiber, through secondary biochemical mechanisms.

Fiber is sometimes considered to be a laxative, but this "label" is misleading. For example, bran (insoluble fiber), when consumed with an adequate fluid intake, can cause a laxative effect. However, certain gel-forming fibers, such as beta glucans from oats or pectin from apples can be used for their balancing effects on digestive function to control diarrhea. Therefore, it is more appropriate to consider fiber as a "modulator" of bowel and other gastrointestinal functions, not just a laxative. One simple issue is clear. To derive the benefits of any type of fiber, the fiber must be taken with liberal fluid intake. Fiber unaccompanied by adequate water intake will "clog" the bowels.

## Fiber is Health Giving

The role of fiber in the diet and health promotion is apparent in many recent scientific studies. The Zutphen study (Kromhout et al., 1982) not only supported the "fiber hypothesis" but showed a relationship between dietary fiber intake and a reduction in death from all causes that were examined in the study. The importance of Zutphen's study has been grossly underestimated in contemporary medical literature. This study was a 10-year prospective analysis of diet and death in 871 middle-aged men in Holland between 40 and 59 years of age. In summary, this research showed that men with a low intake of dietary fiber had about a three times greater risk of death from all causes than men who had a high intake of dietary fiber. Of major importance was the clear observation that the risk of death from a variety of causes seemed to decline with an increasing intake of dietary fiber. The Zutphen study indicates that a diet rich in fiber (of the order of about 35 g/day) is protective against death from several chronic disease, especially heart disease.

There is always a problem in projecting a cause and effect relationship from studies of populations and diet (epidemiological studies). In the Zutphen study other factors may have operated in addition to diet, including issues such as exercise, cigarette smoking, pollution, and psychological factors. Urbanization and a rise in socioeconomic level in Western societies have signaled the onslaught of several preventable chronic diseases. The characteristics of an individual's diet seems to be pivotal in retarding this disease onslaught.

## Fiber is Metabolized in the Colon

Dietary fiber is widely acclaimed in the media and medical literature as possessing general health benefits. Fiber has been called "unavailable carbohydrate", since it contains complex polysaccharides that are not a significant energy source because of their lack of digestion and assimilation by the body. A minor amount of energy is derived from certain fibers in the form of absorbed fatty acids (SCFA). Plant fiber is delivered into the colon (large bowel), where it is metabolized and fermented by bacteria to produce volatile fatty acids (SCFA), gas and energy. These SCFA (acetate, butyrate and proprionate) are absorbed into the body and they have very favorable effects on body chemistry involved in the combat against Syndrome X (vide infra).

The delivery of the fiber to the colon is very important in understanding the effect of fiber on human physiology. First, most types of fiber are hydrophilic (adsorb, absorb, and retain water), and they produce bulk for the colon to exert its actions. As previously mentioned, this bulk assists in normalizing motor function and "bulks" up the stool. People who consume a high-fiber diet have softer, more voluminous stool than those who consume a low-fiber diet. Fiber can alter the normal bacterial populations present in the large bowel, and it can promote the growth of more friendly type of bacteria. Thus, fiber is prebiotic i.e. it provides food for friendly bacteria to grow (probiosis).

The generation of fatty acids (SCFA) and gas from the colonic fermentation of fiber explains why there may be a temporary and often unpleasant period of time when the colon adapts to an extra fiber load. Fatty acids derived from the metabolism of fiber by bacteria may promote frequency of bowel action and excessive gaseousness. Frequency of bowel actions and excessive flatus are common during the early stages of introduction of a high-fiber diet. These effects may be welcomed by many people who are constipated. However, many people may fail to comply with a high-fiber diet if they are not prepared to withstand an early phase of "gastrointestinal adaptation". Consuming a high fiber diet is often a physiological shock to most Westerners, many of whom tend to have contracted, constipated colons that produce small, hard stools. The simple solution is to introduce extra fiber in the diet in a gradual manner and remember that the discomfort caused by any extra fiber load is often only short-lived.

## How Much Fiber?

The optimum daily intake of dietary fiber has not been defined and needs may vary from person to person. What type of fiber? How much? And How Often? are questions that have led to different and sometimes confusing answers. Defining the amount of fiber intake as a proportion of the total daily caloric intake is problematic. It is suggested by many nutritionists that for every 2500 calories consumed in the diet about 30 grams of fiber should be taken, but needs vary by age and type of fiber consumed. For example, most studies show that only soluble types of fiber will affect blood fats (cholesterol) to a major degree (see, beta glucans in soluble oat fiber, later in this section).

Table 44 shows the many benefits of fiber for health but it is the water soluble types of fiber that are of great significance in the combat against Syndrome X. A very important and complex study of the health benefits of fiber showed that oat fiber (soluble form) improved blood lipids (Ripsin CM and colleagues, JAMA, 267, 3317-3325, 1992). The most important findings in this study was the characterization of the beta glucan fraction of the soluble fiber as an active component of oat fiber. Earlier studies had shown that as little as 3 grams of certain fractions of soluble fiber from oats (beta glucans) could reduce blood cholesterol levels and this effect was most obvious in people with the highest blood cholesterol levels. In other words, the higher the initial cholesterol level the greater the cholesterol-lowering effect. Furthermore, the cholesterol-lowering effect seemed to be dose related meaning that two or three doses of 3g or more of beta glucans from oats would magnify the cholesterol lowering effects.

| Effect of Fiber | Comment |
|---|---|
| Satiety | Studies by the author and others have shown that the bulk provided by fiber can cause a sensation of fullness by distending the stomach and slow |

ing the rate at which
stomach emptying occurs.

Slowing stomach emptying

The rate at which food is delivered from the stomach to the
intestines controls the rate of
absorption of many
substances, including glucose.

Altered absorption in the
small intestine

Soluble fibers form viscous gels
which can interfere with
the absorption process in the
small bowel in a positive (e.g.
slows glucose absorption) or negative manner (e.g. blocks
calcium absorption). Delaying
glucose absorption results in
lower peak blood sugars and
reductions in surges in insulin
secretion – an ideal effect in the
combat against Syndrome X.

Lowering of blood lipids

Blood cholesterol is lowered by
several mechanisms (see
Table 45). Beneficial effects
occur on different blood fats
(lipoproteins e.g. VLDL). Reduced
cholesterol synthesis in
liver occurs and reduced chy
lomicron formation.
(micelles blocked)

Beneficial effects on the
lower bowel

Fiber is fermented to short chain
fatty acids (SCFA) which
provide energy for cells lining the
colon and exert other
beneficial effects in the body.
Fiber dilutes toxins in the
bowel, lowers the pH of stool,

promotes healthy function of lining cells of the colon and regulates bowel actions.

Intrinsic Metabolic Effects of Soluble Fiber (IMEF)

Beta glucans are fermented by bacteria in the colon to short chain fatty acids (acetate, butyrate and proprionate). Proprionic acid enters the liver from the colon and inhibits enzymes that cause the synthesis of cholesterol (HMG CoA reductase). Thus, the IMEF of beta glucan is to work, in part, like a "statin-type""cholesterol lowering drug (HMG CoA reductase inhibitor). Short chain fatty acids from soluble fiber may regulate appetite and have other beneficial effects.

**Table 44: A summary of the major benefits of soluble fiber.**

## OAT FIBER EMERGES FOR SYNDROME X

Much interest has focused on the ability of soluble fiber from oats to lower blood cholesterol. This information has been the focus of widespread media advertizing to support the use of oat containing breakfast cereals. Fiber derived from oats has also been shown to lower blood cholesterol levels when added to a low-cholesterol, low-fat diet. Furthermore, people with significant elevations of blood cholesterol have been shown in clinical trials to have reduced their blood cholesterol with the addition of soluble oat fiber to a fat-reduced diet. Although whole forms of oat soluble fiber lower cholesterol, it has been recently discovered that the most active component is a special fraction called the beta glucan (glucocolloid) component of oat soluble fiber (G. Inglett PhD, USDA, Patent 6,060,519). This effect is demonstrable with as little as 7.5 g of the 10% beta glucan (glucocolloid) component of oat fiber per day and this component of oat fiber is available in supplements and functional foods e.g. (X-Trim, Cardio-X, Xenotrol, MetrimX, X-Connection, X-Smoothie, X-Nutrition and Bravo flavored milks etc.)

How does oat fiber lower blood cholesterol? Unfortunately, the answer to this question is not fully understood. Some clues to the cholesterol-lowering mechanism of oat soluble fiber emanate from studies in animals, where comparisons of blood lipids were made on different types of oat-derived soluble fiber. Soluble oat fiber diets protects some animals from early atherosclerosis, due to reduced cholesterol absorption. It causes increases in bile acid secretion by the liver, or decreases bile acid pools by an indirect effect of adsorption and stool bulking. Increasing stool bulk may cause the elimination of cholesterol and bile acids from the intestine, thereby preventing their reabsorption into the body. Even more complex factors operate in reducing cholesterol, including effects on the metabolism within the colon or changes in body hormonal responses. The SCFA, generated from the fermentation of soluble fiber in the colon, especially proprionic acid, play a role in these blood cholesterol lowering effects of soluble fiber (vide infra).

Many studies show soluble fibers, such as those found in oats (oat soluble fiber) apples (pectin) or beans (guar), to be generally more effective at reducing blood cholesterol levels than insoluble fibers. This role of soluble fiber in decreasing cardiovascular risk has been grossly underestimated. In a review of the lipid-lowering ability of fibers, Dr. James Anderson MD and colleagues (1986) reported several controlled scientific studies that indicated that oat bran or beans in the diet can reduce cholesterol by 19%, whereas, guar, pectin and psyllium supplements in the diet can lower cholesterol by 8%, 15% and 16%, respectively. These findings imply that a diet that is high in fiber content is a very useful adjunct to promote cardiovascular wellness and oat derived soluble fiber is preferred for this purpose. More recent data on the administration of the beta glucan, patented-fraction of soluble oat fiber show remarkable reductions in blood cholesterol, in some cases equivalent to those observed with a cholesterol-lowering drug (25% reductions).

The fiber content of beans, some fruit, carrots and a variety of cereals have been shown to lower cholesterol when incorporated into the diet. Much attention has focused on the superiority of oat bran as a particularly valuable controller of blood cholesterol. In one study, healthy volunteers who were following the dietary guidelines of American Heart Association (AHA) were split into two groups one month after initial diet induced a lowering of blood cholesterol. One group received oatmeal supplements and one did not. It was determined in this study that the group receiving oatmeal experienced significant reductions in blood cholesterol over and above those induced by the AHA diet, compared with those who did not consume oatmeal (VanHorn, 1988).

## Oat Soluble Fiber Emerges as a Real Alternative to Cholesterol–Lowering Drugs

The efficacy of oat bran is impressive and, like soy protein, it has been proposed as a real option to avoid drug therapy in the control of high blood cholesterol. Doctors Kinosian and Eisenberg (1988) performed an important study that examined oat bran as an alternative to drugs for treating high blood cholesterol. This study looked at the cost-effectiveness of oat bran versus two prescription cholesterol-lowering drugs (colestipol and cholestyramine). In this study, oat bran was perceived as more cost-effective than these drugs with a conclusion that this natural option may be preferable to drug therapy. Whilst more potent lipid-lowering drugs have emerged since this study was performed in 1988, there is no reason to reject effective natural options to lower cholesterol, especially given the isolation of beta glucan extracts of soluble fiber from oats that have versatile, safe and potent effects on blood cholesterol-lowering.

## Revisiting the Mechanism of Action of Soluble Fiber and Beta Glucans from Oat Fiber

The precise mechanisms that account for the ability of soluble fibers, especially fractions of oat fiber, to lower blood fats are still under investigation. The ways in which beta glucan and other soluble fibers work are summarized in Table 45. It is likely that several mechanisms of action of fiber are indirect. For example, it is known that high blood sugar can cause high levels of insulin in the blood. High blood insulin levels can stimulate the enzyme systems that cause bad types of cholesterol to be manufactured by the liver. The enzyme in question (3-hydroxy-3-methylglutaryl Coenzyme A, or HMGCoA reductase) is stimulated by insulin and inhibited by "statin type" cholesterol-lowering drugs. Thus, one can see just how valuable soluble fiber is as an alternative to taking an expensive "statin drug" that has a worrisome side effect profile. In fact, recent studies show that "statin drugs" are best reserved for "high cardiovascular risk" or diabetic patients and I propose that soluble fiber and especially beta glucan soluble fiber fractions from oats are the first line option. This option is rooted in science and logic and it has nothing to do with definitions of "alternative" or "conventional" medicine.

| Action of Fiber | Comment |
| --- | --- |
| Slows stomach emptying | Slowing stomach emptying "smooths out" rises in blood glucose and insulin which reduces cholesterol synthesis in the liver (a key issue in Syndrome X). |
| Inhibits digestive enzymes | The gel formed from soluble fiber "protects" some food from absorption e.g. fats absorbed in packages called micelles. Micelles are needed for fat, cholesterol and bile acid absorption. These provide substances that form chylomicrons which transport fat in the blood stream. |
| Inhibits mixing of digestive juices, stops enzymes breaking down fats | Soluble fiber binds bile acids and inhibits other absorptive functions starch and protein, with a reduction in energy transfer functions (calorie intake). |

| Colonic fermentation | The production of the SCFA pro prionate in the colon results from fermentation of soluble fiber. Proprionate is absorbed and it inhibits HMG CoA reductase, the enzyme that stimulates cholesterol synthesis in the liver. |
| --- | --- |

**Table 45: How does soluble fiber lower blood cholesterol or balance blood fats?**

FIBER AND BLOOD GLUCOSE REGULATION

Diabetes mellitus is often associated with multiple risk factors for cardiovascular disabilities and deaths, such as obesity, hypertension and high blood cholesterol. Extracts of soluble oat fiber (beta glucans) have an ever increasing role to play in controlling these risk factors. Beta glucans function to control body chemistry that is altered by insulin resistance and diabetes mellitus. Several researchers have suggested the use of oat soluble fiber or other soluble fibers as an adjunct to the management of diabetes mellitus and increasing numbers of physicians are applying this approach. In early experiments, it was shown that the addition of oat (and other soluble fiber) to a drink containing 100 g of glucose reduced post-prandial (after meal) hyperglycemia (high blood sugar) and hypoglycemia (low blood glucose). Thus, soluble fiber was able to smooth the absorption and delay the metabolic incorporation of ingested glucose into the body. This work has been followed by more definitive studies in which the addition of oat fiber to test meals significantly lowered the blood glucose levels at periods after eating. In addition, certain types of blood lipids (especially triglycerides) were reduced at intervals after the test meals.

Considerable evidence supports the facts that soluble fibers normalize bowel function, lower blood lipids, and assist in control of blood glucose levels. Soluble oat fibers can help to avoid both high or low blood sugar in specific circumstances, in part, by their effects on modulating glucose absorption. This effect smoothes out blood glucose swings and, in turn, reduces surges in insulin secretion. For these reasons, certin soluble fibers (pectin or guar gum) and extracts of soluble fiber (e.g. beta-glucans) are very valuable at controlling the adverse circumstances of glucose intolerance (insulin resistance). Insulin resistance is the hallmark of Syndrome X and soluble fibers from oats are emerging as one of "Mother Nature's" versatile answers to the problem.

## Beta Glucans Stimulate Immune Function

Beta glucan is a complex polysaccharide (carbohydrate) that is found predominantly in yeast (Saccaromyces cerevisiae), cereal grains (oat and barley) and several life-forms including: mushrooms. Beta Glucans have been used in alternative medical practice to enhance immune function, promote wound healing and lower blood cholesterol.

There are polysaccharide receptors on certain immune competent cells and it is believed that certain dietary polysaccharides (beta glucans) stimulate or "prime" their activity. All glucans are made up of simple sugars (e.g. glucose) linked together in various chemical configuration. Glucans from different sources tend to have a different linkage pattern of simple sugars. For example, yeast derived glucan is a 1,3/1,6 linked molecule, whereas the glucan from maitake mushroom has a reverse in this chemical configuration.

In the early 1980's, Dr. J.K. Czop and Dr. K.F. Austen defined the presence of a receptor for beta glucan on human monocytes and studied its action (J. Immunol, 134, 2588-93, 1985). When beta glucans bind to the macrophage (monocyte) receptor they induce several functional changes. The macrophage tends to increase its phagocytic ability and release several cytokines (e.g. interleukins such as IL-1 and-2). This triggers other cells, such as T lymphocytes, to exert their function. One added mechanism of action of beta glucan is believed to be a significant antioxidant effect.

There have been several studies with beta glucan in animals and humans that show a clear benefit of this polysaccharide on balancing or stimulating immune functions. For example, in one study, the feeding of yeast derived supplement containing beta glucan to victims of severe trauma resulted in a six-fold reduction of hospital acquired pneumonia. Several uncontrolled, clinical observations suggest that beta glucan may be a valuable cough and cold (flu) preventive and it may have a beneficial effect on wound healing, by presumed immune- modulating mechanisms. The benefits of taking beta glucan have been most apparent with high daily dosing (at least 750 mg/day).

## GET THE RIGHT TYPE OF CARBOHYDRATE

A diet that has a relatively high content of complex carbohydrates is somewhat protective against cardiovascular disease. One must distinguish the difference between simple sugars that cause rapid swings in blood glucose compared with complex carbohydrates that are assimilated more slowly by the body. Complex carbohydrates are often accompanied by fiber in the diet. One key study that dictates the importance of selecting complex carbohydrates and fiber is the Ireland-Boston-Diet-Heart Study, reported in 1985. In this prospective (forward looking) study, over a twenty year period, the diets of three groups of individuals were analyzed and subsequent causes of death were surveyed about 23 years later.

The analyses showed that dietary cholesterol intake and the ratio of saturated to unsaturated fats were higher in those with coronary artery disease, but the individuals who did have coronary disease tended to have much less total complex carbohydrate and fiber intake in their diet. In this study, the researchers concluded that the dietary difference that accounted for the increase in coronary heart disease was most likely more related to a decrease in the intake of complex carbohydrates rather than a change in the intake of dietary fat. Whilst some proponents of the Glycemic Index (see later) tend to question the advantages of complex sugars versus simpler sugars, their benefits are obvious, if only because of their sources in fiber-rich food, which have a low glycemic index!

## REFINED SUGAR: SIMPLE SUGARS

The role of refined sugar consumption in the causation of cardiovascular disease has received considerable attention in the scientific and lay press. Refined sugar (sucrose or fructose) exerts a number of undesirable effects on the body's metabolism, including: increased tissue damage by oxidative mechanisms, inhibition of immune function and interference with vitamin C transport. Excessive dietary intake of simple sugars "flogs" the pancreas to secrete insulin by gyrating blood sugar and it plays a role in the cause of type 2 diabetes mellitus. Prompt increases in blood triglycerides occur following a sugar-laden meal and even acute alterations in immune defenses in the body are noted (decreases in white cell function). Several arguments have surfaced that dietary elimination of refined sugar and the incorporation complex carbohydrates, soluble fiber and selected micronutrients in the diet may prevent or reverse cardiovascular and other degenerative diseases. Certainly, this approach will have a favorable impact on the components of Syndrome X.

## How Soluble Fiber Slows Down Sugar Absorption

As research focussed on the versatile health benefits of soluble fiber over the past decade, new discoveries have provided the basis for a revolutionary approach to the nutritional management of cardiovascular risk factors within Syndrome X. In the 1970's, researchers proposed the dietary addition of soluble fiber to improve blood sugar control in people with established diabetes mellitus and in individuals with a tendency to low blood sugar (hypoglycemia). In essence, it was discovered that soluble fiber could reduce or "smooth out" the rise in blood sugar and insulin that is experienced after the intake of sugar, especially simple sugar (Holt S et al, Lancet, 1, 636-9, 1979).

To understand these effects, one needs to review the basics about glucose tolerance. As sugar (glucose) is rapidly absorbed into the blood stream, the blood sugar rises rapidly and insulin is secreted to push glucose into cells for energy production. Scientific studies performed by my colleagues and I in the mid 1970's showed that this effect of soluble fiber could be explained by a reduction in the rate of sugar absorption into body (Holt S et al, Lancet, 1, 636-9, 1979). The reduction in the rate of absorption of sugar was related in part to the rate at which the sugar was presented to its site of maximum absorption in the small intestines. In this process, the rate limiting step is the rate of the emptying of stomach contents (food) into the small intestine, where most things are absorbed.

In simple terms, the sequence of events concerning the role of fiber in preventing rapid and high peaks in blood glucose can be summarized.

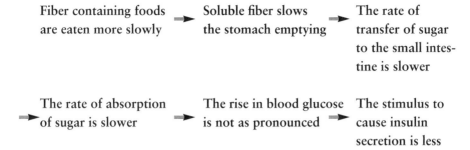

These simple events are very important in the combat against Syndrome X, where rapid swings in blood sugar cause compensatory increases in insulin secretion (hyperinsulinism). High blood insulin levels (hyperinsulinism) in the presence of insulin resistance is at the root of the cause of obesity, high blood cholesterol, high blood pressure and cardiovascular disease in Syndrome X.

The "magic" of soluble fiber is related, in part, to the simple notion that it slows down sugar absorption. This phenomenon of slowing sugar absorption is, in my opinion, the most common basis of the Glycemic Index, a concept that has "revolutionized" the design of many modern diets. The Glycemic Index has relevance in overcoming Syndrome X and other health problems, but it requires some reappraisal in terms of understanding the mechanisms of action that operate to constitute the "proposed concepts".

## THE GLYCEMIC INDEX

The "Glycemic Index" is a phenomenon that we shall continue to hear more about in the future. In simple terms, the Glycemic Index is a way of describing the ability of different foods to cause a rise in blood sugar. Foods laden with simple sugars can be expected to cause a rapid rise in blood glucose to high levels and, as such, they are the prime examples of foods with a "High Glycemic Index". It is possible to rank foods in terms of their Glycemic Index. In fact, foods can be given a Glycemic Index Score, by comparing the effects on blood glucose in comparison to a reference food such as pure glucose. The Glycemic Index has been described as a groundbreaking medical discovery that should guide dietary choices for wellness promotion. Whilst the Glycmeic Index is a useful concept, it is not novel or new. Its role in planning diets for health and weight loss has been emphasized in a dozen recent books, but the concepts may have been "hyped" to a level which transcends a basic knowledge of nutritional science. I propose that the concept of the Glycemic Index can be interpreted, in major part, in terms of simple gastrointestinal physiology that was well documented prior to the description of the "Glycemic Index".

## SIMPLIFYING THE CONCEPT OF THE GLYCEMIC INDEX

We are aware, in simplistic terms, that slowing down sugar absorption slows down the rise in blood sugar and reduces the peak levels in blood sugar that are achieved following sugar intake. Again, I stress that one major rate limiting step in this whole process is the rate at which the stomach empties its contents into the small intestine. It is inside the small intestines where the vast majority of nutrients, including glucose, are absorbed into the body.

In the book "The Glucose Revolution" (Hodden and Stoughton, London, UK, 1998), Dr. Anthony Leeds MD and colleagues provide a painstaking analysis of foods in terms of their Glycemic Index. In addition, these authors attempt to characterize the factors which influence the Glycemic Index of a food. I propose that many of the principal factors that decrease the Glycemic Index of a food are those which tend to slow the emptying of the stomach. When Dr. Leeds and his colleagues list physical or chemical factors of food or their fiber, sugar or fat content, there is an important omission in explaining that these factors are most often those that affect the rate at which the stomach empties. Studies of my colleagues and I have shown that many factors affect the rate at which the stomach empties which, of course, will alter the measured Glycemic Index. For example, the size, constituents, temperature, pH, osmolality of meals or food, all affect the rate at which the stomach empties its contents; as does any disease state, change of posture, drug therapy etc. (Holt S, Gastric Emptying, Control and Measurement, Survey of Digestive Diseases, 3, 4, 210-229, 1985).

## DIABETES ALTERS STOMACH EMPTYING:
## WHERE THE STORY GOES WRONG!

Diabetes mellitus can be complicated by a slowing of the rate of stomach emptying. This is an unfortunate complication of diabetes mellitus that acts in a way to defeat the benefits of slowing of stomach emptying with soluble fiber or "watching" the Glycemic Index of foods. Slowing of gastric emptying is a negative effect of established diabetes mellitus on the nerves and controls that regulate the movements of the stomach. This condition is called "diabetic gastroparesis" (gastro=stomach, paresis=paralysis). In this condition, the rate at which the stomach empties is often grossly delayed. This delay in stomach emptying can cause major problems in control of blood sugar in diabetic individuals and adding fiber to the diet or focussing on foods with a Low Glycemic Index is no longer a valuable or predictable approach in such individuals.

## THE GLYCEMIC INDEX IS NOT THE WHOLE STORY

Just as I believe that the Glycemic Index of food is not the whole story in the combat against Syndrome X, alterations in stomach emptying is not the whole story of how soluble fiber improves glucose control, lowers cholesterol and helps with weight control. The concepts of Glycemic Index and altered stomach emptying "stand up" in circumstances where one measures their effects at specific points in time (acute effects), but the relevance of this whole story to what happens over a period of time with repeated intake of food is more dubious (chronic effects).

This situation has led to the proposal that soluble fibers exert metabolic (body chemistry) effects independent of their effects on Glycemic Index or the slowing of sugar absorption by delaying stomach emptying or the slowing of glucose absorption in the small bowel. The "intrinsic metabolic effects" of fiber (IMEF) have only recently begun to be understood.

## THE INTRINSIC METABOLIC EFFECTS OF FIBER (IMEF)

Whilst the administration of soluble fiber at the same time as glucose (sugar) administration slows glucose absorption, it became apparent that soluble fiber given over a period of time cause beneficial changes in sugar absorption which could be measured independent of the simultaneous administration of soluble fiber, long term soluble fiber administration could itself cause improved glucose tolerance (*sugar absorption curves) without the simultaneous (at the same time) administration of the soluble fiber. Animal experiments also showed material changes in the absorption of substances (nutrients and even drugs with chronic fiber closing), independent of the presence of the fiber at the time of testing.

How soluble fiber causes these effects is beginning to be understood. There appears to be an intrinsic (internal) metabolic effect (effect on body chemistry) of soluble fiber (the IMEF). To understand this intrinsic metabolic effect of soluble fiber, one must re-examine its far reaching effcts on several body strucures and functions (Table 46).

| Effect | Comment |
|---|---|
| Fiber containing foods have to be chewed, stimulate saliva flow | Works against "rapid eating" which can result in enhanced calorie intake. |
| Delays the emptying of the stomach | Soluble fiber tends to "dilute" the contents of food and slows the emptying rate of the stom ach. Its presence can enhance satiety by stimulating stretch receptors in the stomach that make people "feel full". |
| Altered intestinal absorption | Soluble fiber can alter transit of material in the small intestine where most nutrient absorption occurs. May interfere with some nutrient absorption e.g. trace metals and calcium. Improvement in blood sugar profiles are seen over time. Intestinal adaptation occurs. |
| Changes in function of large bowel | Soluble fiber tends to promote the growth of friendly types of bacteria in the colon which, in common with fiber itself, can have a major impact on health through beneficial effects on |

| | |
|---|---|
| | cancer risks, immune function, elimination of dietary toxins etc. Fiber regulates bowel habit. |
| Production of short chain fatty acids (SCFA) | SCFA are produced by the fermentation of fiber in the colon. These SCFA are beneficial to functions of the lining of the bowel and they may act to help glucose and cholesterol balance in the body —a systemic effect. |

**Table 46: Effects of soluble dietary fiber on body structures and functions.**

Of all effects of soluble fiber, I stress their role in the production of short chain fatty acids (SCFA) in the colon as being of particular importance. These SCFA are produced by fermentation in the right side of the colon mainly and they include acetates, proprionates and butyrates (all acids). These acids are small in size and they are readily absorbed from the colon in the veins that drain into the liver (portal veins). The liver is the seat of cholesterol synthesis. Evidence suggests that the SCFA may exert favorable effects on bile acids which are involved in cholesterol synthesis. Components of soluble fiber cause bile acid excretion to increase in the stool and blood cholesterol levels tend to fall.

The SCFA can be absorbed into the body and they have some documented beneficial effects on glucose metabolism. Increases in SCFA levels, produced by fermentation of soluble fiber in the colon, can cause a reduction in blood sugar levels following meals. These changes in blood glucose handling in the body do not occur by simple mechanisms in humans, but SCFA appear to be able to improve both glucose tolerance and insulin sensitivity (combat insulin resistance). It is believed that the effects of SCFA on glucose balance may be a function of the SCFA of "acetate types" derived from soluble fiber. In contrast, the cholesterol lowering effects of soluble fiber may be more related to the generation of the SCFA of "proprionate types". This oversimplification of the biochemical actions of SCFA has not reached a consensus opinion in the scientific literature.

It is noteworthy to reiterate that beneficial effects of soluble fiber on blood cholesterol and sugar can also occur by their simple effects on the viscosity of food. Sticky fiber is slow to move through the upper digestive tract, but it is relatively fast moving through the lower digestive tract. Whatever, the precise mechanism of action of soluble fiber, one of the most important contributions of the use of fiber for health comes from the work of the USDA agricultural chemist, Dr. George Inglett PhD who has unlocked "the secret of soluble fiber".

## DR. G. INGLETT AND THE "SECRET OF SOLUBLE FIBER": BETA GLUCANS FROM OATS

Real advances in the application of soluble fiber fractions for health comes from the unlikely source of chemical food processing. In May 2000, Dr. George E. Inglett PhD of the USDA was awarded a patent for isolating components of soluble fiber, made up principally of beta glucans. This important research has resulted in the development of components of soluble fiber that form a colloidal suspension with water (beta glucan-hydrocolloids). These hydrocolloids are very palatable, can act as fat replacements in the diet and can be added to foods to make them functional for health; or they can form the basis of valuable dietary supplements or functional foods (e.g. X-Trim, Cardio-X and Xenotrol etc.). These glucocolloid, beta glucan components of soluble fiber have several health benefits which can be prominently summarized:

- Beta glucan, hydrocolloid components of soluble fiber can be used as a saturated fat substitute in foods and drinks.
- Beta glucans, hydrocolloids can lower total blood cholesterol, lower triglycerides and work to increase levels of good cholesterol (HDL).
- Beta glucans, hydrocolloids have a very low glycemic index and they help blood glucose control, in part by overcoming insulin resistance?
- Beta glucans, hydrocolloids can assist in weight control by promoting satiety.
- Fractions of soluble fiber, including beta glucans, have cancer preventive benefits.
- Soluble fiber can lower the risk of heart disease and secondarily through weight loss and partial control of insulin resistance it can indirectly lower blood pressure.

- Soluble fiber improves gastrointestinal function by producing a healthy environment in the colon with growth of friendly bacteria and the production of metabolically active SCFA.
- Soluble fiber (beta glucans) have an antioxidant function that is complemented by other components of fiber.
- Beta glucans have some putative, beneficial actions for the management of inflammatory bowel disease, irritable bowel syndrome, gestational diabetes, polycystic ovary syndrome (PCOS), non-alcoholic fatty liver disease (NAFLD) and other disorders.
- Beta glucans and other soluble fibers have versatile IMEF (intrinsic metabolic effects) expressed in part by the actions of fermentation products (short chain fatty acids, SCFA) produced in the colon. The benefits of the generation of SCFA are wide ranging.

### RESEARCHERS CONFIRM THE BENEFIT OF OAT SOLUBLE FIBER

I have stated earlier that these are many studies that confirm the versatile health benefits of oat fiber. Even in the 1960's oat fibers were shown to lower blood cholesterol (de Groot and colleagues, Lancet, 2, 303-4, 1963) and more recently research has shown that people who consume beta glucan fractions of oat fiber can lower their risk for hypertension, glucose intolerance (diabetes) and obesity – combat Syndrome X!

Not all health practitioners realize that beta glucans have their own antioxidant actions. These antioxidant actions of fractions of oat fiber may reduce damaging oxidation of dietary fats by a factor of 80%.

A striking benefit of soluble oat fiber (beta glucan) addition to the diet is its ability to be substituted for fats (fat substitute) in the diet. It is fats that often provide excess calories. This makes the beta glucan component of fiber an ideal ingredient for use in functional foods.

Because the "fat-taste-preference" of Western society is very difficult to overcome. It can now be appreciated that the fractions of soluble oat fiber (beta glucan, hydro colloids), isolated by Dr. Inglett, are tailor-made to combat Syndrome X. Every cardinal feature of Syndrome X is counteracted variably by the isolated beta glucan (hydrocolloid) component of soluble oat fiber which lowers cholesterol, secondarily lowers blood pressure, controls weight and helps to overcome insulin resistance; with the overall effect of reducing coronary heart disease and the added benefits of cancer prevention. The patented hydrocolloid (beta glucan) fraction of soluble oat fiber together with other soluble fibers are one of the most important nutritional discoveries of the 20th Century which will have widespread application in the new millennium (see www.combatsyndromeX.com, www.syndromeX.cc www.themetabolicsyndrome.com and www.syndromeX.tv, in Spanish www.sindromeX.com).

## COMPARING SOLUBLE FIBERS WITH "STATIN" CHOLESTEROL LOWERING DRUGS

Research has highlighted the favorable effects of soluble fiber on blood lipids (cholesterol and lipoproteins). I have mentioned that the most important clinical study on the effect of soluble fiber from oats on blood cholesterol was reported in the Journal of the American Medical Association in 1992, by Dr. C.M. Ripsin and colleagues. This study showed that the reduction of blood cholesterol achieved was related to the amount of soluble taken, but individuals with the highest blood cholesterol levels showed the most significant cholesterol lowering effect. This is a very important observation that has not percolated completely into medical practice, where a tendency exists to jump to the use of a "statin" or other drug when cholesterol levels are in the very high range. I believe that those individuals with very high blood cholesterol form a group that represents an "absolute indication" for the use of oat soluble fiber extracts, given the documented beneficial effects of this type of fiber. In addition, the same benefit exists with the use of soy protein for cholesterol-lowering.

It has been demonstrated that the cholesterol lowering effect of oat fiber is particulary related to the beta glucan water soluble fraction of "oat bran". Whilst the precise mechanism whereby fractions of soluble oat fiber reduce cholesterol is still underexplored, recent studies show that these effects are not merely related to the physical properties of soluble fiber such as viscosity and nutrient binding properties. Fractions of soluble fiber from oats seem to have major effects on the formation of low density lipoproteins in the liver and there may be an effect on fat transport particles (chylomicrons) generated in the small intestine. Whilst the effects of soluble fiber on chylomicon production are likely due to the physical properties of fiber, the effect of soluble oat fiber fractions on LDL formation in the liver are due to a metabolic effect (the IMEF).

To further review the key to understanding how soluble oat fiber interferes with LDL production one must examine our knowledge of the fate of this fiber in the digestive tract. We have learned earlier that the soluble fiber is fermented by bacteria in the colon to produce a group of chemicals called short chain fatty acids. Each of these fatty acids (SCFA), derived from fermented fiber, have specific effects on key aspects of body chemistry.

To reiterate the actions of SCFA is unimportant. The two most important types of short chain fatty acids are acetate and proprionate. These acids are absorbed into the body and they pass through the main veins draining the digestive tract towards the liver. When proprionic acid (proprionate) enters the liver, it inhibits enzymes that form LDL (low density cholesterol, bad cholesterol). The enzyme system inhibited by propionate from fiber is called HMG CoA reductase which is the enzyme inhibited by "statin- type" drugs (e.g. Lipitor, Zocor etc.). Whilst this biochemical action of proprionic acid has been debated, it is well documented in experimental animal research.

The major difference in the action between proprionate from oat soluble fiber and statin drugs is that the fiber derived proprionate inhibits HMG CoA reductase without the side effects of the drugs. Thus, the intrinsic metabolic effect (IMEF) of soluble fiber gives a statin "drug like" effect without side effects and its actions are more versatile than cholesterol lowering drugs, due to its other beneficial actions on mechanisms that control blood cholesterol (e.g. alteration of bile acid chemistry, blocking absorption of cholesterol precursors, interference with micelle formation etc.).

## OTHER TYPES OF SOLUBLE FIBER AND THEIR FRACTIONS

Pectin, guar gum and soluble fiber from cereal grains all possess advantages for use in individuals with Syndrome X. Current research has focused on beta glucan fractions of soluble fiber which appear to have specific advantages in blood cholesterol reduction, blood glucose control and appetite suppression. Soluble fiber forms a good substrate to encourage the growth of friendly bacteria in the colon and probiosis (the feeding of friendly bacteria) is associated with many health advantages, including reductions in blood cholesterol. Friendly bacteria grow particularly well in the presence of prebiotic substances such as soluble fiber and related substances called fructooligosaccharides. Some new forms of fructooligosaccharides have been shown to exert beneficial effects that may be useful in Syndrome X. In addition, there are components of legumes (beans) which may help balance blood glucose. There may be other, undiscovered fractions of legumes which can help blood glucose regulation. One recently described extract of white kidney beans (Phaseolus vulgaris) seems to have a modest effect on lowering blood sugar and this effect is not due to the fiber content of the bean, but it is related to the presence of a compound called Phaseolamin.

## TECHNICAL NOTES (FOR HEALTHCARE GIVERS)

The fiber hypothesis generated by Dennis Burkitt MD in the 1960's was based largely on epidemiological investigations. It stimulated a great deal of scientific work to attempt to explain why such an apparently "inert" substance (fiber) would have such wide ranging health benefits. Sorting out "types of fiber" resulted in arguments among basic scientists about the various physico-chemical properties of fiber; at least until the basic distinction between the health effects of soluble and insoluble fiber was somewhat clarified.

Impressed by the resemblance of hydrated soluble fiber (guar, pectin, soy, oat and mixed legume soluble fiber) to "liquid concrete", I was stimulated to examine the effect of soluble fibers on the emptying rate of the human stomach (Holt S et al, Lancet, 1, 636-9, 1979). The work of my colleagues came at a time when Dr. David Jenkins MD and his associates had reported the effects of soluble fiber on "smoothing out" post prandial blood glucose levels; observations that had importance for the nutritional control of diabetes mellitus, "dumping" following gastric surgery and the subsequent coining of the terms Glycemic Index (Jenkins).

Much of my work in the 1970's had been directed to examine the correlation between the rate of drug or nutrient absorption and the rate at which the stomach empties. This relationship had been of particular interest to several members of the Department of Therapeutics at the University of Edinburgh. Quite simply, the rate at which the stomach empties its contents into the small bowel (the site of maximal absorption of most substances) will determine substance absorption rate, especially if a compound is freely diffusable through the walls of the small intestines. Of course, in the mid 1970's when my colleagues and I performed the research on gel fiber, the intrinsic metabolic effects of fiber (IMEF) were still largely a focus of debate.

The work of my colleagues and I showed that stomach emptying rate was more important in many clinical circumstances than hitherto supposed. Slowing the absorption of drugs (especially those with a short half life, T-1/2) can result in therapeutic failure and even slowing the rate of alcohol absorption can result in less inebriation during acute alcohol intake. However, several researchers including my colleagues and I had postulated the presence of an "intrinsic metabolic effects" of fiber (IMEF), especially soluble fiber. Thus, it was believed that fiber caused biochemical adaptations independent of its physicochemical properties (e.g. viscosity). It was the work of chemists, most notably George Inglett PhD, that resulted in the isolation fractions of soluble fiber that could be studied for their intrinsic metabolic effects (IMEF), perhaps the most important of which is the production of SCFA, especially proprionates, in the colon, and their role in cholesterol-lowering.

Scientists still wrestle to explain the far reaching consequences of dietary fiber intake for health, but simple effects of soluble fibers on gastric motor function appear to be one of the most important operants. Effects of soluble fiber on gastric function goes a long way in explaining the "modern concept" of "Glycemic index" which is neither novel nor new, especially if one traces the early development of the "story of soluble fiber" and its untold "secrets".

It would be misleading to consider soluble fiber from oats as the only example of health giving soluble fiber. Other types of fiber share properties in common with soluble fiber from oats, but none have been used to date commercially in extract form, focusing upon the active beta glucan component. Valuable types of soluble fiber for Syndrome X include apple pectin, citrus fruit pectin, guar gum, soluble fiber from soybeans and other legumes. Several studies have demonstrated that multiple forms of soluble fiber have cholesterol lowering effects and blood glucose balancing effects following meals. Of particular interest is the emerging use of extracts of rice bran. Recent studies show that specific fractions of rice bran may have potent cholesterol reducing properties. However, rice bran is not as versatile as oat bran for use in functional foods because of its distinctive flavor and it does not have the same appealing mouthfeel that soluble oat fiber extracts possess. Rice bran is, however, a very efficient source of water soluble fiber because more than 90% of the total fiber content of rice bran is water-soluble. Commercial forms of soluble fiber that are commonly used as bowel regulators e.g. psyllium and ispagula husks are not as efficient as oat soluble fiber in lowering cholesterol, balancing blood glucose or promoting satiety, for the "feel full weight loss trick".

## CHAPTER SUMMARY

Medical, nutritional and chemical sciences have defined the active constituents of soluble fiber (beta glucans) that work to counteract the components of Syndrome X. Whilst a consensus in the actions of beta glucans may not exist, the beta glucan fraction of soluble fiber from oats can reduce blood cholesterol, secondarily lower blood pressure, help control obesity and variably overcome glucose intolerance. Referred to as "the secret of soluble fiber" in the title of this chapter, the application of this "new", natural, substance can play a major role in the combat against Syndrome X (please see www.combatsyndromeX.com). However, many other types of soluble fiber may be beneficial for Syndrome X.

# NATURAL OPTIONS FOR SYNDROME X AND CARDIOVASCULAR HEALTH

## NATURAL PRODUCTS REQUIRE "NEW PARLANCE"

When discussing the prevention or treatment of disease, the Governments of many countries stipulate that "drug approval" is required. A good example of a "drug claim" is the statement of "lowering blood cholesterol," for which "drug approval" is perceived to be mandatory. In 1994, the Federal Government passed legislation in the form of the Dietary Supplement and Health Education Act (DSHEA), which permitted the use of limited claims of health benefits for natural products (dietary supplements), but such claims are not to be confused with drug claims, at least at law.

As a consequence of this legislation (DSHEA), health claims for supplements are often stated in "veiled" or "couched" terms. These terms are often neologisms and amount to "closet drug claims". In the case of blood-cholesterol-lowering, the DSHEA permits expressions such as "maintenance of a healthy blood cholesterol", but it will not allow a claim of "lowers blood cholesterol" for a dietary supplement. I stress that most of the remedies of natural origin that I describe in this section of the book are dietary supplements and "drug claims" cannot be made to describe their actions.

Unfortunately, the reader who is not familiar with the legalities of pharmaceutical or supplement claims is often confused by this situation. The situation has been explained as a circumstance where a dietary supplement can be described as having an effect on a body structure and function, but not on a disease. This has created a troublesome "enigma" of modern medicine, especially as food or supplements become increasingly used as "medicine". Consumer surveys imply that people use dietary supplements most often with the intent of preventing or treating disease. This use is directly contrary to the law (in the US), but who would be foolish enough to really believe that medicine should or could be legislated? As more physicians select remedies of natural origin, treatment matters become quite complex for the healer and the patient. This enigma of modern medicine should be resolved.

Whilst I must make the situation quite clear in terms of the law, I stress that the inability to make a "drug-type-claim" with a remedy of natural origin does not necessarily mean that no evidence exists for its benefit. In fact, the evidence for the health benefits of many dietary supplements is increasing and it can be communicated in third party literature, provided such literature is geographically separated from the "product" (dietary supplement) in question. This "geographic separation" of third party literature from dietary supplements can occur in retail locations, but not in electronic format on the world-wide web.

Where I discuss a branded dietary supplement, I mention the name only to highlight that scientific support exists for that "form" of natural product. Readers must be aware that dietary supplements of the same class may differ materially in composition and presence or absence of "active ingredients". I referred earlier to "me too" drugs, and I highlight that the dietary supplement industry is replete with "copy-cat products", except the "cats" are often very different. This situation must prompt "caveat empeator", when it comes to shopping for dietary supplements (nutraceuticals or bio-pharmaceuticals or genomeceuticals or any other "ceuticals")

## APPLYING NATURAL MEDICINES

Simple, gentle and effective approaches to general health exist within the framework of natural medicine. Nutritional, botanical and herbal approaches to maintain cardiovascular health and combat Syndrome X have taken a diminutive, second place to drugs for the management of hypertension, glucose intolerance, high blood cholesterol and cardiovascular disease. This situation causes a mix of a "appropriate" and "inappropriate" pathways of disease management. Whilst we recognize the clear benefits of new pharmaceutical approaches to disease, one must balance this approach by the knowledge that the initiation and progression of Syndrome X is related to adverse lifestyle and "environmental hazards", often created by humankind. A lifestyle problem is amenable to lifestyle change and it may not require a "lifestyle drug". "Lifestyle drugs" are a new and nebulous fad. Several theories which focus on nutritional lifestyle in the causation of heart disease are summarized in Table 47.

| Theory | Comments |
| --- | --- |
| Cholesterol Theory | Convincing evidence implicates hyper-cholesterolemia as a major risk for cardiac disease. However, the cholesterol theory is incomplete and when applied alone as the treatment objective, it may be ineffective. |
| Triglyceride Theory | A good correlation exists between blood triglyceride levels and coronary heart disease. Triglycerides increase with high saturated fat and refined carbohydrate diets. |
| Sugar Theory | Simple sugars raise triglycerides, increase oxidative damage and have other adverse metabolic effects. Very important issue in Syndrome X where insulin resistance operates. |
| Oxidation Theory | Oxidized cholesterol and triglycerides damage arterial blood vessels. Fruit and vegetables contain antioxidants e.g. ellagic acid, anthocyanidins, flavonoids |
| Deficiency Theory | Deficiency of one or more essential nutrients, e.g. vitamins, minerals, essential fatty acids, may raise blood cholesterol, cause oxidative and stress heart disease. |

| | |
|---|---|
| Vitamin Theory | Linus Pauling proposed a unified theory to explain the cause and cure of cardiovascular disease with vitamin C. The deficiency of vitamin C may result in the deposition of repair proteins in arteries. Other vitamins and minerals carry clear benefits in CVS disease e.g. vitamin E, selenium, marine coral minerals etc. |
| Syndrome X | Obesity, hypertension, high blood cholesterol and insulin resistance aggregate to form a silent killer. Insulin resistance is the real miscreant. Refined sugar is a major cause. |

**Table 47** : The principle nutritional theories or concepts of the causation of coronary artery disease are listed with relevant comments. The Cholesterol Theory is not the whole story (see Section 2, Combat Cholesterol) and each other theory is somewhat incomplete.

The answer to a lifestyle related disorder, such as Syndrome X, is not a drug or a surgical operation, but it is primarily a lifestyle change (see Section 6). Several remedies of natural origin may be ideal to incorporate into lifestyle programs to combat Syndrome X. We have explored the pivotal role of soluble fibers, especially beta glucan extracts of soluble fiber in Section 7. The issues are not complete without consideration of other potentially effective natural or nutritional approaches to cardiovascular health (or Syndrome X). A number of dietary supplements (nutraceuticals, nutriceuticals) of herbal, botanical or nutritional origin may be of value and this chapter provides a short summary of the use of remedies of natural origin for cardiovascular health. For a more detailed discussion of some of these issues, readers are referred to my earlier book "The Natural Way to a Healthy Heart" (S. Holt MD, M. Evans Publishing Inc., NY, NY, 1999).

## VITAMINS

A great deal of research exists on the role of vitamins in the prevention or treatment of cardiovascular disease but much of the data are conflicting.  Few healthcare givers would argue with the concept that antioxidant vitamins (beta carotene or vitamins A, C and E) or selected antioxidant phytonutrients (phyto=plant) could exert beneficial roles in allaying atherosclerosis and heart disease, but much emphasis has been placed on the B vitamin niacin because of its demonstrated cholesterol lowering ability.

Niacin in high doses (2-3 grams per day) has been shown to lower cholesterol and it may reduce the risk of myocardial infarction (heart attack) and death.  However, niacin has unpleasant and significant side effects, including: distressing "flushes", liver damage, flare-up of peptic ulcer, precipitation of gout and even impaired glucose tolerance. These side effects have limited the  use of niacin as a cholesterol-lowering treatment.  Niacin use in high dosages for lowering cholesterol should always be undertaken with medical supervision.  One serious limitation of high dose niacin therapy is its relative contraindication in patients with diabetes mellitius.  In this situation, niacin may cause poor blood sugar control and increases in serum uric acid.  Thus, high dose niacin therapy often disqualifies itself for the management of Syndrome X, where glucose intolerance exists. Niacin is a natural substance and it serves to illustrate the important point that "natural" does not always mean "safe". Furthermore, it appeals to "Paracelsian leanings", where it is proposed that everything is toxic, it is just down to the dosage amounts !

Several other vitamins have been shown to exert a beneficial effect in the treatment or prevention of atherosclerosis.  In this regard, vitamin C and E may have a special role and much of their benefit is ascribable to their antioxidant effects (Table 48). However, high dose vitamin therapy in people with established cardiovascular disease should be undertaken with medical advice only.

| Vitamin | Effect on Atherosclerosis |
|---|---|
| Niacin | Lowers LDL, total cholesterol and raises HDL but has side effects. |
| Folic Acid | Supplementation may reduce plasma levels of homocysteine, an atherogenic amino acid. |
| Vitamin B6 | B6 deficiency in animals results in atherosclerosis. Blood B6 levels fall in myocardial infarction and supplementation of B6 may inhibit platelet aggregation and prolong clotting time. Used with folic acid to lower blood homocysteine levels. |
| Vitamin C | Blood and leucocyte C levels are decreased in atherosclerosis. Cholesterol-7-alpha-hydroxylase is vitamin C dependent. Vitamin C stimulates lipoprotein lipase and is required to hydroxylate proline. |
| Vitamin B12 | Deficiency of B12 raises homocysteine levels which fall with B12 supplements. |
| Vitamin E | Plasma levels of E are lower in heart disease. Supplement may increase HDL, prevent oxidation of LDL, reduce the size of a myocardial infarct, inhibit platelet adhesiveness and stimulate endothelial repair. Very high doses of E (greater than 5 times RDA) are not recommended except under close medical supervision. |
| Vitamin D | Animal studies show some deleterious effects of high doses of vitamin D on blood vessels. Not recommended as a primary supplement for cardiovascular health. |

Table 48 : A summary of the putative role of some vitamins in the prevention or treatment of cardiovascular disease (coronary heart disease or atherosclerosis). Readers with established cardiovascular disease are referred to obtain the advice of a nutritionist or naturopath or medical practitioner because of the potential danger of adverse effects from some types of excessive vitamin intake.

## PANTETHINES FROM PANTOTHENIC ACID (VITAMIN B5)

Pantethine is derived from the B vitamin pantothenic acid and it has been used in Japan for more than thirty years as a pharmaceutical for the safe treatment of blood lipid disorders. This vitamin derivative is converted by the body to co-enzyme A which plays a major role in lipid metabolism. Some studies suggest that it may improve insulin sensitivity and glucose tolerance and it has predictable antioxidant effects.

Pantethine has become available recently in several dietary supplements but its cost benefit is not determined and its advantages over general vitamin B complex supplementation is not clear. Recent studies highlight the value of vitamin B supplementation in individuals at increased risk of heart attack due to raised blood levels of homocysteine (Tice JA and colleagues, J.A.M.A., 9, 286, 936-43, 2001). Thus, certain B vitamins provide control of both blood homocysteine and cholesterol, but conventional medicine has not focused much attention on correcting high blood homocysteine levels.

## MINERALS

The role of mineral supplementation in the prevention or treatment of cardiovascular disease is still somewhat unclear. Some micronutrients that promote free radical reactions and lipid peroxidation, such as iron and copper, may be relatively contraindicated as supplements in people with heart disease. High levels of body iron stores can be assessed by a blood test (serum ferritin). Recent research published in the American Heart Journal (February, 2000) indicates that high levels of body iron may be related to cardiovascular disease (atheroma) and serum ferritin levels tend to rise with aging in both men and women. Excessive dietary iron intake may play a negative role in the progression of Syndrome X.

In contrast, calcium and magnesium are essential for normal contractile function of the heart. Table 49 summarizes some of the information on minerals and atherosclerosis. In recent years, we have learned a great deal about the value of mineral supplementation in the presence of overt or marginal mineral deficiency. The recognition of the versatile and potent benefits of mineral micronutrients has led to increasing use of colloidal or chelated minerals, e.g. coral calcium or marine coral minerals.

| Minerals | Effect on Atherosclerosis |
|---|---|
| Calcium | Ca can decrease total cholesterol and triglycerides and (Ca) deficiencies or excesses of Ca can promote atherosclerosis. It is believed that Ca within cells is involved in atheroma formation. |
| Copper (Cu) | Cu deficiency is associated with high blood cholesterol and decreased HDL. Cu is toxic in high doses. |
| Iron (Fe) | Fe may contribute to atheroma formation. |
| Chromium (Cr) | Cr supplements may raise HDL and lower total cholesterol and LDL. Deficiency of Cr is a risk factor for arteriosclerosis. |
| Magnesium (Mg) | Mg deficiency is more common than recognized. It can result in an increased risk of coronary disease, sudden cardiac heath, heart attack and abnormal heart rhythm. |
| Selenium (Se) | Low blood levels of Se predispose to atheroma. |
| Zinc (Zn) | Zn blood levels may be reduced in atherosclerosis. It may exert both beneficial and untoward effects on blood lipids. Zn helps insulin function. |

**Table 49**: A summary of some of the effects of minerals on atherosclerosis. Self-medication with large doses of minerals is not advised in the cardiac patient.

# A Pot-Pourri of Nutritional Agents for Cardiovascular Health

There are a large number of nutrients that have interesting but underexplored effects on atherosclerosis and related forms of cardiovascular disease. Among the most important are antioxidants and omega 3 fatty acids (vide infra). The effects of some of the many nutrients on atherosclerosis are summarized in Table 50.

| Nutrients | Effect on Atherosclerosis |
| --- | --- |
| L-Arginine | Supplementation may assist endothelial function in blood vessels. Wide range of benefit. |
| N-Acetylcysteine | Administration has been reported to reduce lipoprotein(a) |
| Aspartic Acid | A nebulous role, may affect Mg+ and K+ balance in cardiac disease. |
| Beta-carotene | May reduce heart attacks in established coronary heart disease. |
| Bioflavonoids | Reduce platelet adhesiveness, antithrombotic. |
| Carnitine | May improve lipid metabolism and has an effect on myocardial energy expenditure. |
| Coenzyme A | Uncertain, beneficial effect on blood lipids. |
| Coenzyme Q10 | Lipid soluble antioxidant with protective effect against atheroma, reduces blood viscosity, cardio-protective. |
| Glycosaminoglycans | Anticoagulant and lipid lowering effects. |

Lecithin                    May normalize blood lipids and reduce platelet
                            aggregation. Effect on lipids is limited and proba-
                            bly related to phospholipid (fatty acid) acid con-
                            tent.

**Table 50:** Miscellaneous nutrients that exert a potential benefit on atherosclerosis and/or cardiovascular disease. In many cases the evidence to
support their use is incomplete (for further information readers are referred
to the book "The Natural Way to a Healthy Heart", Holt S, M. Evans
Publishing Inc., NY, NY, 1999).

## Red Yeast Rice: Effective But Contentious?

Red yeast rice (Hongqu, Monascus purpureus) contains a substance
called mevinolin which acts like a "statin-type" drug by blocking the enzymes
involved in the synthesis of cholesterol in the body (HMG CoA reductase). It
has been marketed in the US as a dietary supplement but it has been the subject of much debate among lawmakers. There are many natural substances
from herbs or botanicals that act like a drug and many prescription drugs
have their basis in plant extracts. Red yeast rice is known to be effective at lowering cholesterol, but it is uncertain if it carries the same risks as synthetic,
statin-type drugs. The contentions that surround the use of red yeast rice highlight the enigma of the blurred boundaries between drugs and dietary supplements.

## Soy for Syndrome X: A Partial "Soylution"

The preoccupation with cholesterol-lowering strategies using
drugs has led to a situation where the important effects of sources
of dietary protein on blood cholesterol levels have been overlooked.
It has been recognized for approximately eighty years that diets rich
in animal protein may promote atherosclerosis and, in contrast, high
vegetable protein diets may lower blood cholesterol and the risk of
cardiovascular disease. The famous nutritional researcher Dr. James
Anderson MD and his colleagues of the University of Kentucky have
reported a collection of studies in the New England Journal of
Medicine in 1995 which showed that soy protein effectively lowers
blood cholesterol. Soy protein and soluble fiber (beta glucan) sup-

plementation of the diet are obvious choices for lowering blood cholesterol by natural means in clinical practice. They can be used together in a diet to combat Syndrome X.

There are several beneficial cardiovascular effects of soy foods that can be explained in a manner independent of their effect on blood cholesterol. They are summarized in Table 51 and a more complete account of the benefits of "soy for health" are to be found in my earlier two books on this subject (Holt S, "Soya for Health", M. Liebert Publishers Inc., Larchmont, NY, 1995 and "The Soy Revolution", Dell Pulishing, Random House, 2000). Recently, the role of soy for health has come under fire and these contemporary concerns about soy require some discussion.

| Fraction of Soybean | Cardiovascular Effect/Benefit |
|---|---|
| Soybean Oil | Fresh oil contains 7% omega 3, 50% omega 6 and 26% omega 9 fatty acids, lecithin, phytosterols. Commercial soybean oil is refined or partially hydrogenated. This destroys some essential fatty acids that are associated with cardiovascular wellness. |
| Lecithin | Made often from soybean oil and contains omega 3 fatty acids. It is a phospholipid with diverse functions on blood lipids and cell membranes. |
| Isoflavones (genistein, daidzein) | Isoflavones have a poorly defined role in cholesterol lowering and possess anti-atherogenic and anti-thrombotic effects. Inhibit LDL oxidation. |
| Soy Protein | Protein of soy origin has a very convincing role in lowering cholesterol and improving blood lipid profiles. |
| Peptides | Peptides in soy may chelate oxidizing elements in the diet and may lower blood pressure in a similar manner to angiotensin enzyme converting inhibitors? |

| Sterols/Stanols | Sterols can lower blood cholesterol by competing with the absorption of cholesterol in the diet. Soybean sterols have emerged as components of functional foods. |

**Table 51:** Fractions of Soybeans with Cardiovascular Benefit

## Defining Aspects of the Soy Controversy

Soy is not a stranger to "roller coaster enthusiasm" for its use, but doubt still remains among some consumers about whether or not soy food is safe or of medicinal benefit. The issues cannot be resolved as long as some protagonists of soy incorporation into Western diets exaggerate claims of benefit and some antagonists take isolated pieces of research, draw misleading conclusions and then apply them as unjustified generalizations. Claims that the soy legume is an inferior source of protein containing antinutrients or toxic components have not been dignified by thousands of contemporary scientific studies that delineate the potent and versatile health benefits of the many components of soy.

Soy food or fractions of the "soya" bean play an increasingly well defined role in the prevention or treatment of a variety of diseases including, but not limited to: coronary heart disease, cancer (breast, colon and prostate), osteoporosis, prostatic enlargement, gallstones, obesity, the symptomatic management of menopause, premenstrual syndrome and Syndrome X. These apparent "panacea" benefits of soy may have been presented occasionally in a misleading way to the average consumer. Such consumers think of "soy" as anything ranging from unhealthy, hydrogenated soy oil in junk food to complex culinary offerings, such as meat substitutes or delicious desserts.

Whilst a preoccupation with semantics often serves little purpose, it is clear that health benefits attributable to soy are only defined by modern research in specific formulations of soy or in certain contexts of its use. To illustrate this issue, the advent of the FDA approved for soy to reduce the risk of coronary heart disease refers only to soy protein intake, in the context of a low saturated fat diet, in a dose of at least 25 g/day. Many health benefits of soy have been ascribed to the isoflavone content of soy, prompting the popularity of pills containing extracted soy isoflavones. Whilst many fractions of soy are health giving, crude soy is not friendly food and it requires substantial processing before it fits the preferences of the Western palate, or before it can be included in natural products. The problem is that some "adulterated" derivatives of soybean processing, such as hydrogenated soybean oil cannot be considered healthful. This reinforces the notion that the synonymity of the words "soy and health" is sometimes in question.

## THE ANTI–SOY MOVEMENT

Whilst several components of the soybean are an ideal candidate for use in "nutraceuticals" and functional foods, soy food seems to offer an environmentally-friendly, alternate source of protein. Considerable scientific epidemiological and experimental evidence exists that the incorporation of more vegetable sources of protein (especially soy) into Western diets could have a major beneficial impact on public health. Unfortunately, many social, political and economic factors operate on the attempts of Western society to move towards greater fruit and vegetable intake. These factors promote the emergence of Syndrome X. Desirable dietary changes of fruit and vegetable enrichment have been defined in the medical literature for seventy years, but they still defy global enactment

Protagonists of raw (non-processed) food or "contemporary", nourishing traditions (meat and dairy products) have recently hammered the health benefits of soy in a merciless manner, often by quoting several misguided interpretations of isolated scientific observations. In the past couple of years, popular publications in the lay, trade and "scientific press", with titles that include exploitive terms such as tragedy, hype, myth and "truth" have begun to sway some public opinion away from the health benefits of soy. The more hide-bound, anti-soy supporters allege that soy does not prevent heart disease by both acknowledging its cholesterol lowering benefit and then denying that lowering cholesterol prevents heart disease. This questionable logic is sometimes found among several, radical, dietetic interest groups, and it serves to create confusion among consumers.

## INADEQUATE KNOWLEDGE PROVOKES SAFETY CONCERNS

The appropriate desires to define safe and effective intakes of soy fractions (e.g. isoflavones) for health and the uncertainty at "pitching" correct estimates have been amplified by some into raging arguments on the potential toxicity of isoflavones. Isoflavones are phytochemicals with estrogen balancing and antioxidant effects. Much precedent exists to consider soy isoflavones in the diet to be safe. Population studies imply their safety, based on thousands of years of use, especially in Asian communities. A massive biological experiment has occurred without planning, where soy is fed in very high amounts to farm animals in the US without untoward effects. No substantive evidence of toxicity exists in humans at levels of total isoflavone intake of 50 mg per day (or higher in my opinion up to 80 to 120 mg/day). Other examples of frank, anti-soy propaganda exist and include statements that soy may increase cancer risk and that modest soy intake can cause hypothyroidism, whilst most data supports the contrary. As blatantly absurd as some of these suggestions are, they sway the more fickle dietary opinion.

## THE FAT/WEIGHT LOSS TREND: SOY TO THE RESCUE

There are some highly conservative, "educational" foundations that cling to the notion that excessive saturated fat intake is consistent with general health. In contrast, several "weight loss gurus" propose liberal fat intake, even in saturated format, as an efficient way to lose weight. Few scientists doubt the importance of balanced essential fatty acid intake, but the cumulative evidence for excessive intake of unhealthy types of fat in the promotion of cardiovascular disease, cancer and obesity is overwhelming.

There may be arguable short term weight loss benefits of high fat and protein intake. The induction of ketosis by severe carbohydrate restriction and increased fat intake induces weight loss as a consequence of early fluid loss, the induction of anorexia and the elimination of carbohydrate as a substantial source of calories in the diet. This dietary approach is associated with cardiovascular risks and other unknown health problems, especially if this dietary approach is applied in a sustained manner. In contrast, certain forms of soy are ideal dietary substrates for weight loss because soy is low in calories, has a low glycemic index and it counteracts many of the problems associated with accelerated weight loss e.g. hyperlipidemia, calcium loss, gallstone formation, and loss of lean muscle mass. For these reasons, soy merits attention as a nutritional antagonist to Syndrome X.

## Fermented or Non-Fermented Soy?

A prevailing opinion exists among some nutritionists that the health benefits of soy are most likely to be delivered when soy is given in a fermented format. Soy has been a dietary staple in Eastern Asia for thousands of years and traditional, soy-based diets are composed often of fermented soy bean products including miso, natto or ancestral-fermented tofu. Much of the evidence for the health benefit of soy in the diet is derived from population studies that compare Eastern Asians on soy rich diets with Westerners on diets that contain more animal protein and refined carbohydrates. These epidemiological studies show that the occurrence of breast or prostate cancer, heart disease, Syndrome X and adverse symptoms associated with the menopause is less in populations consuming soy. In many circumstances the type of soy consumed in these populations is of the fermented variety.

This line of reasoning to support only the use of fermented soy for health is not entirely convincing because processed fractions of soy, such as isolates of soy protein, have been shown in modern, well controlled, scientific studies to have measurable health benefits. The real advantage of soy fermentation is the partial digestion of protein and carbohydrate components of this legume. Enzyme inhibitors within soy are often denatured, removed or neutralized by fermentation. Furthermore, fermentation eliminateds unabsorbable carbohydrate fractions of soy that cause digestive upset, such as abdominal gas and bloating.

Recent research on the absorption and biodisposition of soy isoflavones shows that these compounds have a greater bioavailability (enhanced absorption) when presented to the gut for absorption in deconjugated form. The conjugated isoflavones genistin, daidzin and glycetin are converted variably to their unconjugated forms (genistein, daidzein and glycetein) by the breaking of the beta glucoside bond during fermentation. Therefore, fermented soy can be expected to present freely bioavailable isoflavones that can be efficiently utilized. Pharmacokinetic studies of soy isoflavones support the notion that unconjugated isoflavones have enhanced systemic bioavailability (in acute dosing), but the relevance of these pharmacokinetic observations with chronic soy intake in the diet is in question.

The story of the change of composition of soy fractions during fermentation is not simple. The various fractions of soy and their chemical make up may vary considerably due to many factors including the nature of starting substrates, agents (yeasts or fungi) used for fermentation and physiochemical factors used in various fermentation processes. Although isoflavones are often present in the soybean seed as beta glucosides, a variable amount of these phenolic compounds have a substitution on the C-6 hydroxyl group of the glucose molecule by a malonyl group. Furthermore, the chemical characteristics of the isoflavones can vary by their location within the seed. For example, the hypocotyl segment of the bean may have greater amounts of malonyl substituted conjugated isoflavones than other sites within the bean.

Examples of the variability in soyfoods as a consequence of biotransformation by fermentation or processing include: a low concentration of malonyl substitution in roasted beans, a reduction of isoflavone levels in tofu because of aqueous processing, higher levels of isoflavones in aglycone (deconjugated, format in tempeh than in soynatto etc.

## The Isoflavone Debate

The confusion surrounding the roles of isoflavones in cancer inhibition and/or promotion is attributable, in part, to the current lack of knowledge about their biological actions. For example, one simplistic and misleading idea about these compounds is that they are "phytoestrogens" with unqualified estrogenic effects. Actually, while isoflavones have an affinity for estrogen receptors, they tend to exert lower levels of estrogenic stimuli to cells than endogenous estrogens (e.g. 17-beta-estradiol). This means simply that isoflavones may serve as a "balancing act" for the effects of endogenous estrogens on body tissues. These observations imply that soy isoflavones can act as a "biochemical adaptogen" or a kind of "biological response modifier", especially related to estrogenic status.

Recent work suggests that soy isoflavones can exert estrogenic effects by altering the metabolism of estrogenic compounds in the body. Isoflavones do not have a consistent pro-estrogenic action, and when they occupy estrogen receptors they can block the action of more potent endogenous estrogens, thereby making their overall effect antiestrogenic, particularly in states of estrogen dominance. However, these circumstances surrounding these potential adaptogenic roles of isoflavones are not simple and require further scientific exploration.

Soy isoflavones may exert anticancer benefits because of their function as potent antioxidants and free radical scavengers. Animal experiments and limited human observations show that isoflavones exert an antiangiogenic effect, which is an important step in cancer pathogenesis (and other chronic diseases). Also, the specific isoflavone genistein can interfere with key enzymes involved in cell proliferation and tumor growth. Various isoflavones inhibit tyrosine kinase and deoxyribonucleic acid (DNA) topoisomerase, which is involved in cellular apoptosis.

Thus, soy isoflavones have potential anticancer effects that act independently of any estrogenic or antiestrogenic activity. Despite uncertainties surrounding the actions of isoflavones, the sale of dietary supplements containing these compounds rose by a factor of approximately 250% in the 12 month period ending October 1999 and then tailed off.

Soy isoflavones appear to be quite safe when used in doses with an existing precedent for safety. However, it is important to note that these safety precedents strictly apply to soy food and not soy isoflavones used in concentrated formats. While it is unlikely that anyone would consume more than a total daily intake of 150 mg of isoflavones, even if he or she ate a heavily soy enriched diet, isoflavone supplements are available in a variety of doses. The complex, beneficial actions of isoflavones make them interesting phytochemicals for use in Syndrome X.

## GENETIC ENGINEERING

The increasing use of genetic modification (GMO) in many crops, including soy, has caused considerable public debate and even acts of ecoterrorism. Although the proposed dangers or advantages of GMO soy are hypothetical, there is much uncertainty about the effect of genetic engineering on the ecology and human health. Genetically modified soy is so prevalent in the US that pure, non-GMO soy is hard to obtain. Emblems and labels appear on supplements that claim an absence of GE soy (non-GMO, non genetically modified organism), but are they really GE free? The answer is that often they are not completely free of GE material! The operative terms are "substantially GE (or GMO) free", in a similar manner to which producers use the terms "substantially equivalent", when discussing the nutrient value and safety of GE soy, compared with non-GMO soy. Of course, the word "substantial" implies more than clever semantics. In the US, we are governed by truth in labeling, but where do we stand with qualified truths?

The more academically inclined food scientist has argued against the use of soy concentrates as nutraceuticals. On a practical basis, the health benefits of soy require monotonous and metered dosing and changing dietary habits in Western society has been a losing game. The nobel suggestion that soy should be included in the diet in natural food format is not a pragmatic way to derive the health benefits of soy for many Westerners. Functional foods and dietary supplements made from soya beans are here to stay and many are potentially valuable in the management of Syndrome X.

Amidst recent concerns about the safety of soy itself, further concerns emerge about our modern adulteration of this valuable food. On balance, evidence exists that soy is very health giving and nutritious. In fact, it is a "treasure chest" of medicinal compounds. It is the archetypical example of "medicalized" food. What a tragedy that we have confused ourselves with clever science, propaganda and misinterpretations of reality about soy for health. One thing is for sure, powerful economic influences may stand in the way of dishing up "soya for health".

## STEROLS AND STANOLS

Sterols and stanols are substances found in several plants, e.g. soybeans. Sterols and stanols bear a chemical resemblance to cholesterol. These substances can block the absorption of cholesterol in the gastrointestinal tract and cause favorable reductions in blood cholesterol. A recent study performed by researchers at the USDA (United States Department of Agriculture) showed that individuals who consumed 2.2 g of sterols esters per day lowered elevations of LDL (bad cholesterol) by an average of up to 18% compared with only up to 8.4% with "low fat" diet.

Several types of sterol and stanol esters are available as dietary supplements or functional food ingredients in "fat-based" foods such as margarine (e.g. "Benechol" and "Take Control") or salad dressings. The recommended daily intake for sterols and stanols to reduce blood cholesterol is at 3.4 grams per day or more in one or more meal servings per day. The Standard American Diet (SAD) usually contains less than 0.25 g of plant sterols per day. Whilst this cholesterol lowering approach with sterols and stanols is novel, it is at best an "adjunctive" approach and I fear that their incorporation into margarine will encourage greater consumption of bread containing refined flour and refined sugar. These are the arch-enemies of Syndrome X!

## NOT ALL FATS ARE BAD:
## THE IMPORTANCE OF OMEGA 3 FATTY ACIDS

Fat is regarded as a "dirty word" by many health conscious individuals. This unfortunate assumption overlooks the importance of essential fats as health giving nutrients and it has contributed partially to a modern dietary deficiency state of essential fatty acids (especially of the omega 3 type of essential fatty acids found in fish oil). This widespread deficiency of omega 3 fatty acids in Western communities has passed unrecognized by many. The role of a diet that is high in saturated fat in the causation of a variety of common killer diseases is quite clear, but the role of certain fats in the promotion of health is still clouded in many peoples' minds. Although there are many fats that cause ill health, there are dietary fats that are obligatory to promote good health (especially essential fatty acids of the omega 3 variety).

There are two important categories of essential fatty acids including omega 6 series and omega 3 series fatty acids. Omega 6 series fatty acids are ubiquitous in the diet and are found to a major degree in vegetables, whereas, active omega 3 fatty acids are relatively confined to marine sources. Omega 3 fatty acids are found largely in fish and marine mammals. There are interesting exceptions, certain legumes, such as soyabeans, contain significant amounts of the "precursor" omega 3 fatty acids (alpha-linolenic acid). The two most important "bioactive" types of omega 3 fatty acids with health giving benefits are eicosapentaenoic acid (EPA) and docosahexanoic acid (DHA). These fatty acids are abundant in fish oil.

## UNDERSTANDING THE CHEMISTRY OF ESSENTIAL FATTY ACIDS

Fats may be solids or liquids. The biochemistry of fats is a complex subject but the main focus of interest is to understand the different types of fatty acids, since this knowledge is a key to the understanding of the health-giving benefit of fat in general. A saturated fatty acid is one in which the bonds between the carbon atoms in the molecule contain a shared pair of electrons to form a single bond. In contrast, unsaturated fatty acids contain double bonds. In broad general terms, saturated fatty acids are found within the "less healthy" type of fats (associated with meat and dairy protein in the diet), whereas unsaturated fatty acids are found within the "more healthy" type of fats (associated with fish and plant protein). In other words, saturated fatty acids occur mainly in food of animal origin, whereas unsaturated fats tend to be found

Stephen Holt

in food of vegetable origin. These oversimplifications of chemistry require further explanation.

## THE ESSENTIAL NATURE OF THE ESSENTIAL FATTY ACIDS

The term essential fatty acid implies that the fatty acid cannot be manufactured by the human body and it must be taken in the diet. If an essential fatty acid is not consumed in the diet a deficiency will ensue in exactly the same way that vitamin deficiencies occur. Only a relatively small quantity of the Western diet contains "active" omega 3 type fatty acids (DHA and EPA). These omega 3 types of fatty acids are found mainly in salt water fish and shell fish of cold water origin. The general importance of omega 3 and omega 6 types of fatty acids in the function of the body is summarized in Table 52. Omega 3 and 6 fatty acids are important precursors of substances that have effects on body functions (lipid-mediators or eicosanoids). Fatty acids are also changed into body hormones called prostaglandins (or eicosanoids) that are involved in inflammation, cardiovascular function and cellular health in general.

- The normal function of the immune system
- Formation of substrates for hormone production and effector properties
- Regulation of blood pressure by involvement in vascular tone and collateral circulations
- Regulation of responses to pain, inflammation, infection and cancer
- Controlling glandular secretions and their composition
- Regulation of smooth muscle and neural function
- Effecting cell membrane structure and mitosis of cells
- Regulation of cell oxygenation and nutrient intake
- Providing energy substrates for key organs

**Table 52:** The protean effects of essential fatty acids, eicosanoids and prostaglandins on body function.

## Tracing the Origin of the Health Benefit of Fish Oils

The health benefit of fish oils has been recognized for a long time and it was first identified in studies of the disease profile of races, such as Eskimos, that ingest large quantities of all types of fat, including omega 3 fatty acids from fish oils. Eskimo populations living under "traditional conditions" have a very high consumption of fat and protein in the diet, but a remarkably low incidence of cardiovascular disease. There are a number of other differences in disease profile between the Eskimo and members of Western society. These differences include a relatively low prevalence of inflammatory bowel disease, arthritis and other degenerative disorders. Unfortunately, contemporary data on the occurrence of disease in Inuit (Eskimo) population shows a shift away from the lower incidence of such disease states. This has occurred coincidental with a move toward a Western type diet and the general introduction of "popular" types of adverse lifestyle. Climb the mountains of Peru or brave the climate of the North West Territories of Canada, soft drinks and fast food advertising "complements" the natural beauty.

## The Health Benefits of Fish Oil

There are a variety of cardiovascular health effects attributed to omega 3 fatty acids including a reduction of LDL cholesterol, inhibition of platelet slickness, lowering of blood pressure, variable reversal anginal pain and protection against sudden death from heart attack. Several authors have drawn attention to the benefit of fish oils in the treatment of rheumatoid arthritis, ulcerative colitis, Crohn's disease, psoriasis, migraine headaches, visual disturbance and even yeast infections.

Recent research has shown that omega 3 fatty acids are effective antidepressants and they may benefit children and adults with attention deficit disorder (ADD). A remarkable recent finding is the ability of omega 3 fatty acids to assist the function of genes that control insulin actions (vide infra). This finding has major implications for the use of fish oil in treating insulin resistance which is at the root of the cause of Syndrome X. The potential health benefits of omega 3 fatty acids are legion. These benefits can be further understood by a basic knowledge of the biochemical functions of essential fatty acids in general.

## THE OMEGA 6 AND OMEGA 3 BALANCE

The ratio between omega 6 and omega 3 fatty acid intake in the diet has been the subject of much interest. The traditional Inuit (Eskimo) diet has a ratio of omega 6 to omega 3 of approximately 1 or less to 1, whereas average Western diets have a ratio of omega 6 to omega 3 of anything ranging from 5 through to 30 to 1. Several dietary changes have been mapped over the past century and it is apparent that over the 150 years the consumption of omega 3 fatty acids has dramatically fallen with a corresponding rise in the consumption of omega 6 fatty acids in the average Western diet. This situation is co-incidental with a dramatic rise in the dietary intake of simple sugars. This striking information has been somewhat overlooked by modern medicine and it must be realized that such a fundamental change in fat content in diet, with a shift from omega 3 to omega 6 fatty acids, will result in a completely different composition of body fat with important health implications, due to changes in the balance of eicosanoid (lipid-mediators) production in the body.

The relative amounts of omega 6 and omega 3 fatty acids in the body varies dramatically depending on the tissue in question. The omega 6 to omega 3 fatty acid ratio in nervous tissue is approximately 1to1, whereas the ratio in adipose tissue deposits is approximately in a range of (between 3 and 7) to (1). On average the ratio of omega 6 to omega 3 throughout most body tissue is about (between 4 and 5) to (1). I believe that an optimal ratio of omega 6 fatty acids to omega 3 fatty acids in the diet should be somewhere between 1 and 5 to 1. At a recent "Consensus" meeting at the National Institutes of Health, many scientists proposed that the omega 3 to omega 6 ratio should be 1:1. Remember, this ratio becomes less important if the co-factors (vitamins of B-series etc.) required for the correct biochemical function of essential fatty acids are not present in the diet and if the diet is not generally well balanced.

## Fish Oil Lowers Cholesterol and Helps Insulin to Work

The ability of omega 3 fatty acids to reduce blood cholesterol and induce beneficial changes in other blood lipids such as lowering triglycerides, reducing levels of LDL and VDL, together with increases in HDL have been well documented. Several studies have shown that long-term dietary supplementation with fish oils may exert beneficial effects on blood lipids and cardiovascular disease. Beneficial effects on blood lipids have been observed in cases of familial high blood cholesterol, in patients with high blood triglycerides, in the suppression of VLDL concentrations in the blood, and fish oils have been shown to attenuate the dietary cholesterol induced rise in blood lipoproteins (cholesterol) in humans. This latter observation implies that fish oils may be beneficial in protecting against rises in blood cholesterol from normal dietary intake of cholesterol. This effect almost certainly operates to lower the occurrence of heart disease and it is most notable in the Eskimo on a high fat diet. Fish oil also reduces the tendency to blood clotting by altering platelet stickiness. This effect of omega 3 fatty acids is advantageous in states of Syndrome X, where there is an enhanced tendency to blood clotting (Section 1).

## Sources of Omega–3 Fatty Acids

I reiterate that there is increasing evidence that there may be a widespread deficiency of omega-3 fatty acids in Western diets. Active forms of omega-3 fatty acids are readily obtained from marine sources such as coldwater fish, crustaceans and marine algae, but several plants elaborate alpha-linolenic acid, the precursor of bioactive omega-3 fatty acids. Whilst fish oil contains the active omega-3 fatty acids eicosapentanoic acid (EPA) and docosahexanoic acid (DHA), the omega-3 precursor alpha-linolenic acid requires conversion to active fatty acids by a desaturase enzyme.

The key desaturase enzyme functions with variable efficiency in different people (interindividual variation), resulting in a circumstance where the precursor (alpha-linolenic acid) of active omega-3 fatty acids may not be consistently or reliably converted into the biologically active forms omega-3 fatty acids (EPA and DHA). To consider plant sources of omega-3 fatty acids as a reliable supply of active omega-3 acids is often questionable, despite rhetoric from the purveyors of plant-derived, omega-3 fatty acid precursor-containing, dietary supplements. For example fish oil is a much better source of omega 3 fatty acids than flax seed.

## CRUCIAL CHEMICAL CASCADES

Understanding the cascade of compounds that are synthesized from essential fatty acids (Omega 3 and 6 fatty acids) is a task for even the most informed healthcare giver. The most common types of omega 6 fatty acids are the precursor molecules linioleic acid and its end products of arachidonic acid and adrenic acid. Arachidonic acid (omega-6) and EPA (omega-3) are the main "intermediary" precursors of hormones and complex compounds called eicosanoids of which the prostaglandins and leukotrienes are common examples.

The eicosanoids signal a wide variety of body functions including blood clotting, inflammation and blood pressure regulation. Linolenate is the omega 3 fatty acid precursor found in some plants, e.g. soybeans, flax and canola, and it can be used by mammalian tissues to generate the eicosanoid EPA, which can be converted to DHA. Eicosapentanoic acid tends to result in the production of prostaglandins of types that are anti-inflammatory and anti-clotting in their actions. In oversimplified terms, EPA (an active omega 3 fatty acid) pushes the balance of production of lipid mediators towards more "friendly" types of eicosanoids and resulting prostaglandins, compared with arachidonic acid (an omega 6 fatty acid). An undesirable shift in eicosanoid production in the body occurs variably in syndrome X and results in Syndrome X, Y and Z...

There is no cross-over between the pathways of metabolism of active omega 6 and omega 3 fatty acids, which are generated from linoleic acid and linolenic acid, respectively. However, the relative amounts of generated eicosanoids do exert complex influences on each other. Thus, the omega 6 and omega 3 fatty acids generate signaling compounds (lipid mediators or eicosanoids) with widely differing properties and actions on body structure and function. When the omega balance is "out of whack", many body functions may change for the worse.

## EPA: THE EMPEROR OF FATTY ACIDS

Much interest has focused on the omega 3 fatty acid EPA (eicosapentanoic acid) because of its vital role in balancing favorable eicosanoid production. The acid EPA is readily converted to DHA, which is found in large amounts in cell membranes, especially in the nervous system and EPA is an effective inhibitor of the genesis of "undesirable" forms of eicosanoids from arachidonic acid. For these, and other reasons, EPA has an underestimated role in the management of Syndrome X, Y and Z...(and other diseases)

There are many genes involved in controlling the body chemistry of fats (lipid metabolism) and sugars (carbohydrate metabolism). The active omega 6 and 3 types of fatty acids (not linoleic and linolenic acid precursors) control the expression of genes that affect lipid synthesis. Active types of omega 3 and 6 fatty acids regulate more than ten different types of genes involved in lipid metabolism or energy production. Of major importance are a group of genetic controls related to specific receptors. (e.g. PPAR or peroxisome proliferator-activated receptors).

Evidence has accumulated that the active omega 3 fatty acid, EPA can favorably affect the PPAR (receptor complex), which is involved in insulin action, carbohydrate metabolism and lipid chemistry. Thus, EPA has emerged as a very important way of combating insulin resistance through its beneficial regulation of certain components of the PPAR receptor. EPA (found in fish oil) appears to be a natural and powerful antidote to insulin resistance and it is a emerging as a first line option for Syndrome X, with its cardinal components of glucose intolerance, hypertension, hyperlipidemia and obesity (see www.combatsyndromex.com)

Omega-3 fatty acids are among the most potent and versatile "biopharmaceuticals" available for the treatment or prevention of many common diseases. The evidence for the beneficial effects of omega-3 fatty acids in cardiovascular disease (e.g. Syndrome X, atheroma, coronary heart disease), chronic inflammatory disorders (e.g. rheumatoid arthritis), Crohn's disease, ulcerative colitis, disordered immune function and the maintenance of central nervous system structure and function (e.g. depression and attention deficit disorder) is increasingly clear. Whilst optimal dosages or contents of fish oil concentrates (e.g. ratios of DHA to EPA) are still being defined, medical practice will see the future introduction of purified, proprietary fractions of fish oil (especially EPA > 50% fractions) as key biopharmaceuticals with wide ranging treatment applications (e.g. Oligomega, Cardiomega, etc).

## BOTANICAL INFLUENCES ON CARDIOVASCULAR DISEASES

Botanical extracts have been used for centuries for the prevention and "cure" of disease. Despite the length of time of use of such agents, relatively few conclusive scientific studies are available to support their applications in the prevention or treatment of disease. The development of pharmaceuticals from plants is the basis of the science of "pharmacognosy" through which modern day synthetic drug therapy was largely developed. More than one-quarter of all current prescription drugs are derived from plants. Table 53 summarizes some contemporary knowledge on the use of botanicals (herbs and plant substances) for cardiovascular disease. A fuller account of herbs and botanicals in the management of cardiovascular disease is found in my book entitled "The Natural Way to a Healthy Heart" (M. Evans Publising Inc., NY, NY, 1999).

| Botanical | Active Ingredient | Effect |
|---|---|---|
| Alfalfa | Saponins | Lowers cholesterol in animals. |
| Artichoke | Cynarin | Alters blood lipids. |
| Goldenseal | Berberine | Protects against cardiac ischemia. |
| Bilberry | Anthocyanoside | Reduces platelet aggregation. |
| Pineapple | Bromelain | Inhibits platelet, aggregation, (protease), vasodilator, antianginal. |
| Turmeric | Curcumin | Antithrombotic in animals. |
| Eggplant | May be Pigment | Inhibits atheroma formation. |
| Fenugreek | Debitterized | Lowers blood lipids. |
| Rice Bran | Ferulic Acid | Lowers cholesterol. |
| Garlic | Allicin and other Sulfur compounds | Lowers cholesterol. |
| Onions | Onion oil | Lowers cholesterol. |

| Ginger | May be ground powder aqueous or ethanolic extract | Inhibits platelet aggregation and may lower cholesterol. |
|---|---|---|
| Mukul Myrrh Tree | Guggulsterones | Improve lipid profile. |
| Hawthorn | Procyanidins Flavanoids | Cardiotonic, improves myocardial function, antiarrhythmic. |
| Khella | Khellin | Dilates coronary arteries and ameliorates anginal pain |
| Malabar Tamarind | Hydroxycitric Acid | Lower cholesterol, inhibits atheroma formation, antithrom botic. |
| Grape Seed Extract and Maritime Pine Bark | Pycnogenols and Mixed Flavonoids | Lower cholesterol, inhibit atheroma formation, antithrombotic. |
| Milk Thistle | Silymarin | Reduces cholesterol. |

**Table 53: A list of botanical products with their putative active ingredi-**
ents that have been used with variable success to combat cardiovascular
problems and atheroma. The author stresses that not all of these botanicals are safe for the treatment of cardiovascular disease and the evidence
to support their use of often weak. Self-medication is not advised.
Readers are advised to seek the advice of a qualified medical practitioner
before using any herbal remedy for established cardiovascular disease.

## Nutraceuticals With Special Effects on Syndrome X or Cardiovascular Risk

In addition to soluble fiber (Section 7), soy protein and fish
oil, several other key nutraceuticals are potentially beneficial for use

in Syndrome X. These are chromium, specific antioxidants (alpha lipoic acid, carnosine) and newly discovered fermented forms of barley grains. The potential benefits of each of these nutraceuticals for Syndrome X require a short overview.

## CHROMIUM

Much interest has focused on the ability of the trace element chromium to regulate blood glucose by its actions on the facilitation of the function of insulin. There is no question that chromium has an important role to play in the metabolism of fats and glucose, but exaggerated claims about chromium supplementation as a weight loss measure are somewhat questionable and "excessive" dosing with chromium for weight loss has some unresolved safety issues.

Population studies show that individuals with "high" levels of chromium in their body may have a lower prevalence of heart disease. The importance of chromium in glucose control has been doubted by some scientists, but it has been suggested that chromium may be an important factor in explaining the difference in the rates of diabetes mellitus and atheroma in different geographic locations. The role of chromium in the regulation of glucose and insulin metabolism is well documented, but chromium has major significance in the regulation of blood cholesterol levels. In fact, several recent studies have indicated that chromium supplementation may result in lowering of blood cholesterol.

## CHROMIUM AND SYNDROME X

Chromium is an essential micronutrient with an underestimated and underexplored role in the management of Syndrome X. Observations in humans show that a deficiency of chromium can result in insulin resistance, glucose intolerance and abnormal blood lipid levels. Despite this knowledge, a number of contemporary scientists will not accept chromium as an essential dietary component. This reticence to accept the importance of chromium exists in the face of many studies that show beneficial effects of chromium supplementation on the variable reversal of abnormal glucose balance (both hypoglycemia and hyperglycemia see www.nutrition21.com).

Recent experiments show that chromium occurs in an active form called "low-molecular-weight-binding-substance", abbreviated to LMWCr. This is a peptide bound form of chromium that can be shown to amplify or enhance the actions of insulin – i.e. it can variably overcome insulin resistance. It seems that chromium in this form works by stimulating the actions of portions of insulin receptors, notably insulin-receptor-protein-kinase activity.

Another intriguing action of chromium relates to its interactions with DNA and RNA (genetic material) in cells. Chromium can be found to be concentrated in the nucleus of cells where it is bound to DNA. This binding produces sites of initiation for the synthesis of RNA (transcription processes), which is the mechanism whereby genes exert their effects on body functions. Elegant research has shown that chromium regulates gene expression. It seems likely that chromium aids genes in expression of their actions to favorably effect glucose and lipid metabolism.

Whilst explanations of the actions of chromium on disorders that form Syndrome X components seem complex, it has been known for several decades that natural substances high in chromium help the function of insulin. The most widely recognized chromium-containing, natural substance is Brewer's Yeast which contains one or more fractions called "glucose tolerance factors". The glucose "balancing" components of Brewer's Yeast have been used by some physicians for many years in the treatment of diabetes mellitus. In Eastern Europe, clinical trials of yeast fermented barley have shown benefit in the management of high blood sugar and cholesterol (see later in Section 8, Barley fermentation products).

Some caution is required with the use of chromium. It is not recommended, generally, to exceed a dose of approximately 1000 mcg per day. Some successful studies of the beneficial effect of chromium on blood cholesterol and other disorders have used much higher doses, of the order of 2,000 mcg per day. If high doses of chromium are used, medical supervision is required. Chromium supplements have become increasingly available and are often added to multivitamin supplements. It is believed that chromium exerts its most potent effects when in the form of picolinate, polynicotinate or with carnosine. The picolinate and carnosine-linked forms of chromium seems to have special advantages.

## Special Forms of Chromium

Chromium is efficiently administered in a form bound with other substances that can facilitate or complement its actions in the body. It is known that the absorption of chromium is assisted by certain compounds, including histidine (an amino acid), nicotinic acid and ascorbic acid. Biotin (vitamin H), a member of vitamin B complex, may be synergistic (additive) in its actions with chromium and this vitamin is known to improve blood sugar control by an effect on stimulationg enzymes in the liver (glucokinase) and a supportive effect on the function of insulin secreting cells (beta cells of the pancreas). The corporation, Nutrition 21 Inc., leads the way in chromium research.

By several mechanisms of action, biotin can help breakdown glucose and assist in increasing the body's sensitivity to insulin. When chromium is administered with biotin, the effects of chromium on the enhancement of glucose uptake by cells, glycogen synthesis by the liver and increases in good cholesterol (HDL) appear to be greater than with either chromium or biotin administered alone, (www.nutrition21.com).

## Vanadium

Several research studies indicate that the micronutrient vanadium may assist in the control of blood sugar by promoting the effects of insulin. Vanadium is a trace element that is included in some supplements used to assist in reducing the amount of insulin used by individuals with insulin-dependent (Type 1) diabetes mellitus. Vanadium is usually taken in the form of vandyl sulfate and it has been shown to exert some benefit in reducing cholesterol levels and blood pressure. There are some unknown safety concerns about the use of vanadium, but the commonest side effect is relatively insignificant abdominal irritation. It is notable that vanadium works to improve insulin sensitivity in individuals with Type 2 diabetes but it does not have an insulin sensitizing effect in individuals who are not diabetic. Thus, vanadium appears to be a supplement that would be best used under the supervision of a physician, because alterations in insulin dosages or the dose of blood glucose lowering drugs, or insulin sensitizing drugs may have to be closely monitored. The safety of the use of vanadium supplements in pregnancy and young children is unknown and best avoided in these circumstances.

## CARNOSINE

Carnosine is a combination of two amino acids, alanine and histidine. It has antioxidant actions that are well documented (see "antioxidant effects" later in this section of the book). The functions of carnosine in the body are beginning to be understood. It may exert important effects on the regulation of certain genes in the body and it is known to regulate sugar breakdown, muscle contractions, stimulate immune function and it binds certain metals (copper, zinc and calcium).

The beneficial effects of carnosine on body metabolism are very important in the combat against Syndrome X. It can inhibit glycation effects (formation of AGE, advanced glycation products that occur in hyperglycemia) and it exerts welcome "antiaging" effects. These desirable effects of carnosine are summarized in Table 54.

| Effect of Carnosine | Comment |
|---|---|
| Inhibits glycation and formation of AGE's (advanced glycation end products) | Carnosine can react with agents that cause glycation - a very important issue in causing tissue damage in diabetes and glucose intolerance. Carnosine combines with carbonyl groups found on AGE and their precursor molecules. |
| Anti-aging effects | Carnosine is found in high con centrations in "long-lived" tissues and it can be shown in the lab to stop aging in certain types of cells. These anti-aging actions |

may be related to inhibition of
glycation, antioxidant actions or
effects on immune function. It
prevents protein cross linking.

**Table 54: The two desirable effects of carnosine which are highly rele-**
vant in the combat against Syndrome X.

The inhibitory effects of carnosine on glycation (production of AGE) makes it a valuable approach to the potential prevention of complications of diabetes (compare with alpha-lipoic acid, reviewed later in this section). Research suggests that carnosine may prevent cataract formation and cardiovascular disease. Other underexplored potential benefits of carnosine include inhibiton of amyloid toxicity in Alzheimer's disease, reversal of body inflammation and certain anti-cancer effects.

## ANTIOXIDANT EFFECTS

Antioxidants star in treatment of Syndrome X and they are molecules that fight damaging free radicals. The term "free radical" is applied to a chemical compound which is essentially incomplete in its structure and highly reactive because of its arrangements of electrical charges. This feature of a free radical is called an electron arrangement. The role of free radicals in the causation of a variety of diseases is well recognized. Free radical reactions result in damage to cell membranes that may cause cardiovascular disease, cancer, and premature aging. The scientific discovery of the importance of free radical pathways in the causation of disease occurred largely as a consequence of improvements in understanding of the effects of ionizing radiation (x-rays or radio isotopes) on a variety of living organisms.

The idea that there are free radicals generated in the body as a consequence of normal body processes such as food assimilation and energy production, or as a consequence of a variety of external influences (pollutants), forms the basis of the "free radical theory". To prevent free radical damage to cells, it is possible to provide drugs or agents in the diet that are sometimes referred to as "free radical scavengers". The body has many "built-in" defenses to deal with free radicals that are generated by metabolic processes or other mechanisms. Free radical scavengers are a class of compounds which are referred to as antioxidants.

Whilst free radical generation is believed to play a major role in the causation of aging, cancer and cardiovascular disease, it is used by cells to assist in body defenses. For example, white cells and other cells involved in immune function may manufacture free radicals in order to kill bacteria or viruses. Although the human body does have a number of natural defenses against free radicals, these defenses can be overcome by excessive free radical loads placed on the body. In this circumstance, antioxidant compounds such as vitamins C, E, beta-carotene, selenium and coenzyme-Q10 and many plant or animal antioxidant compounds (phytonutrients, phytoantioxidants) can exert a major beneficial effect, by "mopping" up free radicals. These antioxidant compounds are a common component of dietary supplements used for the prevention and treatment of cardiovascular disease by an increasing number of physicians.

Oxidized cholesterol (LDL) that is formed by free radical damage tends to be deposited in arterial vessels and antioxidants can assist in mitigating this event. However, antioxidants can also act to prevent the occurrence of thrombosis (blood clots) that superimpose themselves on atheroma in the coronary arteries and cause heart attacks. Modern theories of the causation of atherosclerosis imply that the cholesterol-containing plaques in this disorder start among "mutated" smooth muscle cells in the middle layers of the arterial wall. It is proposed by some that this mutation of the muscle cell occurs as a result of free-radical injury. There are many potential sources of free radicals to cause this injury, including components of cigarette smoke or environmental pollutants. These explanations form the rationale for the use of antioxidants in heart disease.

## FREE RADICALS DAMAGE TISSUES

Several types of "free radical" damage occur to body tissues. These include damage to cell membranes (lipid peroxidation), cross-linking of structural and functional proteins, damage to cellular structures (e.g. lyzosomes) and the accumulation of pigments (lipofucsin). This damage can disrupt body chemistry and cause specific damage to walls of arteries. These changes may be variably inhibited by the use of antioxidants in the diet. Neutralizing (quenching) free radicals (e.g. superoxides, hydroxyls, lipid peroxides and hydrogen peroxide) can prevent cardiovascular disease (atherosclerosis), cancer, chronic inflammatory disorders and antioxidants can assist in slowing down the process of body aging. In Syndrome X, a large part of the damage and progression of the disorders are related to free radical damage.

## Oxidative Injury and Coronary Artery Disease

The protagonists of the "free-radical theory" of many chronic diseases have within their midst a few "radical thinkers". This type of lateral thought is to be commended and not dismissed lightly. Increasing evidence has emerged that accelerated oxidative injury is very important in the cause and progression of atheroma and arteriosclerosis. The appeal of these theories is that oxidative damage is amenable to antioxidant therapy which is presumed to have the ability to reverse this damaging oxidative stress to tissues.

The biochemistry that underlies the pathways of free-radical damage to tissues is highly complex, but the principles of oxidative theories are relatively simple. We know that a free radical is a highly reactive but incomplete molecule that is a natural end-result of energy-producing reactions in the body. Some of these free radicals are able to destroy important chemical compounds in the body such as enzymes and proteins.

Extensive damage to cells can occur by the generation of a chain of chemical events by free radicals. Several types of damage can be ascribed to free radicals, as summarized in Table 55. Antioxidants are a diverse collection of nutrients that can stop free-radical damage. Antioxidants, such as vitamin A, beta-carotene, vitamin C, vitamin E, selenium, pine bark extract, coenzyme Q-10, bioflavonoids, anthocyanidins, ellagic acid, astaxanthins etc. can all interfere with free radical-generation and the effects of free radicals. However, some of these antioxidants are not readily available to body tissues to exert a benefit.

- Damage to cellular membranes which protect all cellular functions
- Cross-linking of protein or DNA molecules. Genes are comprised of DNA which can result in mutations
- Lipid peroxidation where fat is attacked resulting in further free radical release
- Damage to cellular lysosomes which contain damaging enzymes

that are released inside cells

- Free radicals cause lippfucsin (age pigment) deposition in cells

**Table 55:** A summary of the types of damage to cells and molecules that can be produced by free radicals.

## Oxidative Stress Prevention: Simplifying Issues

Many individuals recognize the health benefits of antioxidants, but some people are confused about how they work or which ones they should take. The word antioxidant means " against oxidation". Oxidative damage (oxidation) involves oxygen and it refers to a constant process in living tissues where reactive types of oxygen (sometimes called "free radicals") combine with tissues to create oxidative damage. Oxidative damage can affect cell membranes and other vital structures that control normal body functions. Whilst we associate oxygen with health in terms of body tissue needs, on occasion oxygen can be present in a damaging form as a by-product of the chemistry of life.

Certain natural substances or nutrients often act as antioxidants with varying strength for binding oxygen. They can compete with each other for free radical binding. This means that antioxidants can vary in terms of their ability to "quench" oxygen " free radicals". Some nutrients can be utilized in the body to promote the synthesis of antioxidant compounds in the body itself e.g. gluathione production. Classic nutrient antioxidants, which work by direct or indirect effects, include beta-carotene, vitamins A, C, and E and selenium or zinc. Vitamin C is a classic antioxidant that is commonly used, but many botanical and herbal products contain complex molecules with antioxidant properties, eg: isflavones from soybeans, flavonoids from fruit and ellagic acid from raspberries or pomegranates. In fact, the claim of a health benefit of many natural products hinges on their antioxidant profile.

The access of antioxidant molecules to variable parts of the body's cells and tissues is important, as is their potency at quenching "free radicals" of oxygen. New terms have emerged when describing antioxidants e.g. ORAC value. ORAC refers of the ability of a substance to engage in <u>O</u>xygen <u>R</u>adical <u>A</u>bsorption (antioxidant action) qualified by a measure of its $\underline{C}$apacity to do this, i.e. ORAC value. High ORAC values should be noted on supplement labels in the future. Combinations of antioxidants are to be preferred, because the use of high doses of a single antioxidant (alone) may not be healthful e.g vitamin C at high doses can actually cause oxidation in a contrarian manner.

## PLANT ANTIOXIDANTS: POLYPHENOLS AND BIOFLAVONOIDS

Flavonoids are one type of naturally occurring polyphenols that are found in a wide variety of plants. In some circumstances, these flavonoids account for some of the colors that are found in a variety of herbs, vegetables or fruits. The overall effect of these polyphenols (bioflavonoids) in humans is to exert a potent antioxidant effect. By this mechanism bioflavonoids are believed to be capable of preventing a variety of diseases, including cardiovascular disease, viral infections and cancer. In addition, these compounds may play a role in the regulation of blood glucose.

There have been many studies that show the health benefits of bioflavonoids, especially in relationship to the promotion of cardiovascular wellness. Some of the most widely researched examples of bioflavonoids include compounds such as hesperidin, rutin and quercetin. These bioflavonoids occur as mixed constituents in citrus fruit, such as limes, lemons and oranges. Hesperidin, rutin and quercetin are known to protect capillary structure (small blood vessels integrity) and they exert an important role in stabilizing cell membranes. In addition, these compounds are known to contribute to lowering of blood cholesterol and they exert an antithrombotic effect (anticlotting action), by inhibiting platelet aggregation.

It has been proposed that anthocyanidins are capable of lowering blood cholesterol and blood triglyceride levels and they are potent antioxidants. Table 56 summarizes the beneficial effects of plant antioxidants on body metabolism and cardiovascular function. Extracts of berries contain powerful phytonutrient antioxidants (anthocyanidins, ellagic acid and bioflavonoids) and these extracts can be used to great benefit in flavoring beta glucan forms of soluble fiber supplements or functional foods (e.g. X-Trim™, Syndrome X Nutritional Factors™ etc., Section 7).

- Facilitate phospholipid metabolism
- Vitamin C helper effects
- Antioxidant effects
- Vitamin E like activities
- Free radical scavengers
- Protein phosphorylation
- Effects on arachidonic acid metabolism
- Potent effects on redox reactions
- Influence gene expression
- Affect calcium ion transport

**Table 56:** Metabolic effects of flavonoids anthocyanidins, ellagic acids and certain procyanidolic oligomers.

## FREE RADICAL DAMAGE TO THE CARDIOVASCULAR SYSTEM

In common with many other organs in the body, the heart is quite susceptible to damage by free radicals, referred to as oxidative stress. Tissue injury caused by free radicals is known to be a feature of a number of adverse cardiovascular events, such as ischemia of the heart muscle and damage to endothelial cells in the lining of blood vessels. Lipid peroxidation as a consequence of free radical activity is a form of chronic oxidative damage that plays a major role in the development of atheroma and arteriosclerosis. In addition, high blood sugar leads to a circumstance in the body where free radical damage is more likely to occur and protein damage results from the reaction of glucose with body proteins, a process called glycation. The reaction of glucose and body proteins result in damaging types of chemicals called "advanced glycation end-products" (or AGE for short). Not only does insulin resistance result in high blood glucose, it results in oxidative stress and tissue damage from advanced glycation end-products (AGE) formed by glucose bonding with protein. Thus, antioxidants are particularly valuable in the management of Syndrome X and I believe that they should be used on a routine basis.

## ALPHA LIPOIC ACID

Alpha lipoic acid (thioctic acid) is an antioxidant that is produced by many living organisms, including humans. It was first identified as a potato extract and it was fully characterized in the 1950's, when its antioxidant potential was defined. In many respects, the advantages of alpha lipoic acid in the management of diabetes mellitus and Syndrome X bear similarities to those of carnosine, although the compounds are chemically quite distinct.

Alpha lipoic acid plays a major role in body chemistry that is involved in the burning of glucose (oxidation) in small structures inside cells called mitochondria. The chemical structure of alpha lipoic acid gives its access to compartments of cells that contain water and fat. Like carnosine, alpha lipoic acid can help regenerate tissue levels of natural vitamin antioxidants (e.g. vitamins E and C).

In several sections of this book, I have stressed the occurrence of oxidative stress to body tissues in individuals with diabetes mellitus or Syndrome X. This oxidation reaction contributes to cardiovascular complications (e.g. atheroma) and it contributes to insulin resistance. There are several studies that indicate that antioxidants such as vitamin E and alpha lipoic acid may improve the body's sensitivity to insulin. The beneficial effects of alpha lipoic acid have been applied in the treatment and prevention of complications of diabetes, especially in Europe, where it is used as a prescription drug in some countries.

In summary, several studies in the past decade have implied that alpha lipoic acid can lower blood glucose and insulin levels in the glucose intolerant individual and it can facilitate the actions of insulin. Favorable responses to alpha lipoic acid in terms of improvements in insulin sensitivity and blood glucose control have been documented with intakes of 300-1800 mg of alpha lipoic acid per day, but lesser amounts may be effective in synergistic combination products. In common with carnosine, alpha lipoic acid reduces glycation (AGE formation), bolsters actions of other antioxidants in the body and it protects the liver from damage.

## Fermented Barley Extracts (GlycoX™)

Researchers in Yugoslavia have been searching for natural "insulin sensitizers" for many years. These researchers were intrigued by the presence in nature of many organisms that use sugar, but do not regulate this use with the hormone insulin. This phenomenon was proposed by scientists as a primitive way of supplying energy to living organisms that pre-dated the evolution of more precise, hormonal controls of sugar utilization in mammalian tissues (with the hormones insulin and glucagon). Biologists looked to yeast organisms (Brewer's Yeast) in their research. Yeast appears to have novel mechanisms of energy production from sugars that do not utilize hormones, like insulin.

Impressed by these concepts, Professor Dusan Vucelic and his basic science colleagues in Yugoslavia collaborated with a group of physicians, led by Professor Radosav Dragojevic, in the study of yeast fermented extracts of various components of cereal grains (barley) on the control of metabolic abnormalities (sugar and cholesterol) in individuals with maturity onset (Type 2) diabetes. Research at the Military Medical Academy in Belgrade, Yugoslavia showed striking results in the control of blood sugar, blood cholesterol and clinical status of individuals with Type 2 diabetes. Studies performed in one hundred patients with Type 2 (maturity onset diabetes) implied that these natural, fermented barley preparations were able to improve blood sugar control and exert very favorable effects on blood lipids as primary or complementary therapy. The overall effects of these fermented extracts of barley grain were equivalent to the actions of biguanide drugs (e.g. metformin), but there were no side effects.

The early drawbacks of this form of natural therapy was the amount of the natural yeast/barley combination that needed to be given to achieve these effects. The required dosage was of the order of 20 to 30 grams per day. Following these early studies, Professor Dusan Vucelic extended his research by defining the active components of the prototype barley/yeast preparation. This new, more refined extract of barley/yeast has been named "glucose metabolism modulator" (GlycoX) and it is under current intensive research to define its efficacy. Preliminary studies, performed by scientists at VanDrunen Farms, in ten individuals with Type 2 diabetes mellitus and showed benefits in glucose control similar to those obtained with a biguanide drug (e.g. metformin). The active components of the natural preparation (named GlycoX™) are being further characterized and these components may be a combination of the glucose regulating contents of yeast (chromium, glucose tolerance factor or perhaps beta glucans) and the presence of bioactive peptides that may directly affect the process of glucose uptake in body tissues. It appears that this natural product may have great potential application in the management of Syndrome X.

It is notable that the clinical outcomes of the use of this natural product (GlycoX™) made from barley and yeast were quite striking. Professor Dragojevic has summarized early results of a prototype product (containing fermented barley extracts) that was marketed in Yugoslavia under the trade name (Diabet™). He reported an overall average blood sugar decreases of 63%, reduction in levels of "bad" cholesterol by 21%, increases of good cholesterol by 20%; and projected reductions in the risk of cardiovascular disease by 45% in people with established Type 2 diabetes mellitus. The Yugoslavian researchers have received some predictable skepticism from the conventional medical community but they are convinced that their approach is a major advance in the use of a dietary supplement (nutraceutical) in the variable correction of insulin resistance and the combat against Syndrome X.

Whilst this "new" natural extract of yeast and barley malt has not undergone extensive clinical trials in North America, there has been a substantial precedent set for its benefits in medical communications in Eastern Europe. The new patented form of this natural extract is being marketed in the US as GlycoX™.

## Policosanol: Sugar Cane Extract

Whilst the negative effects of excessive dietary sugar are reinforced constantly, its origin in sugar cane is ironic given the identification of policosanol, derived from sugar cane, as a natural agent that lowers blood cholesterol in individuals with Type 2 diabetes mellitus. Policosanol is a mixture of alcohols (higher, primary aliphatic compounds) that can be isolated from sugar cane wax. Much research has been performed with policosanol in Cuba and Central America where it is reported that this natural extract can lower LDL, lower VLDL, increase HDL and decrease triglycerides in humans to a variable degree with apparent safety and lack of drug interaction potential.

## Herbs and Botanicals Regulate Blood Sugar

Several herbs have been used in traditional medical practices to "treat" diabetes mellitus. Some botanical extracts have significant effects on lowering blood sugar and their mechanism of action is not entirely clear. There is a possibility of serious interactions between herbs that lower blood glucose and drugs (antidiabetic medications) used for the same purpose. It is important to use potent herbal or botanical remedies only with the supervision of a healthcare giver that is skilled in the management of diabetes mellitus. Given the increasing use of these remedies of natural origin, each requires a brief review.

## BITTER MELON (MOMORDICA CHARANTIA)

Known by many names (balsam pear, karela, bitter gourd), bitter melon has been described as an "insulin mimic" which seems to lower blood sugar only when blood sugar is elevated, at least in experimental animals! Several human clinical trials performed on the Indian subcontinent imply that bitter melon can decrease the absorption of sugar and enhance glycogen stores in the liver, with an added benefit of modest lowering of blood cholesterol.

Bitter melon can be taken as a specially prepared drink or in supplement tablets or capsules that often contain dried bitter melon combined with other herbs that may regulate blood glucose. Few physicians in Western communities have experience with the use of this botanical and the optimal doses required for a desired response are not clear. The advice of an Ayurvedic physician, naturopath or master herbalist is recommended with the use of "anti-diabetic" herbs or botanicals.

## FENUGREEK (TRIGONELLA FOENUM–GRAECUM)

Used for many years in Ayurvedic medicine, fenugreek powder has been described as effective at balancing blood glucose and reducing blood cholesterol. It appears to be a safe botanical and it is a popular food ingredient in Southern Europe and Asia.

## GARLIC (ALLIUM SATIVUM)

Garlic has been studied extensively for its benefits in cardiovascular disease but results of some studies show inconsistent benefits. This problem may be related to the type (extract or whole) and amount of garlic used. Overall, garlic and other members of the onion family of plants may exert benefits in reducing blood cholesterol and in some cases they may help balance blood glucose.

## Corosolic acid (Lagerstroemia speciosa or Punica granatum)

Corosolic acid is most often used as an extract of Punica granatum, due to the protection afforded the pretty flowering plant Lagerstroemia which grows in China and the Phillipines. This botanical extract has an inconsistent effect on lowering blood glucose levels and optimum doses have not been established.

## Stevia (Stevia rebaudiana)

Stevia is used as an "non-approved" artificial sweetener, but it is worthy of special consideration for use in individuals with Syndrome X. The sweetness of stevia is valuable in "functional" beverages, but this herb may have an added advantage of reducing blood glucose. The dried leaf of the stevia plant taken in large doses (5 grams three or four times a day) has been shown to lower blood glucose in healthy individuals by uncertain mechanisms. More research is required to assess this apparent combination of benefits of Stevia as an alternative sweetener and blood glucose "balancer". Stevia has become a very contentious issue with regulatory agencies who do not consider it to be a safe sweetener, based on some animal toxicity studies. Stevia is not considered "GRAS" (generally recognized as safe) food ingredient, but it can be used in dietary supplements provided that claims are not made.

## Gymnema sylvestre

This bitter tasting herb has been used widely in Ayurvedic medicine to treat diabetes. Clinical trials using Gymnema have reported benefits in lowering blood sugar in people with Type 2 diabetes, in comparison with placebo medicines. There are few comparisons of the use of the herb Gymnema with anti-diabetic drug therapy, but Ayurvedic physicians extoll its superiority to drug treatments. More research is required to define the described effects of Gymnema on balancing glucose, lowering cholesterol and reduction of AGE (advanced glycated protein formation) in Type 2 diabetes.

## Miscellaneous botanicals

Many other herbs and botanicals have been proposed as potential treatments for glucose intolerance and some possess the added advantage of cholesterol control. Table 57 summarizes the potential benefits of some of these agents.

| Herb/Botanical | Actions/Benefit |
| --- | --- |
| Tinospora cordifolia | Inhibits conversion of glycogen to glucose and may reduce cholesterol. |
| Pterocarpus marsupium | May provide inconsistent glucose balance and improve symptoms in Type 2 diabetes. May have an effect on regenerating beta cell (pancreas) activity due to catechin content. |
| Azadirachta indica | An adaptogen with variable benefit on sugar control. |
| Ficus racemosa | May be valuable for weight loss, variable glucose control. |
| Aegle marmelose | Of questionable benefit. |
| Syzygium cumini | Antioxidant components may help diabetes by AGE prevention |
| Cinnamonum tamala | Recent research shows great promise for components of cinnamon to control blood sugar. |
| Atriplex halimu | Reports of improved glucose tolerance in Israeli studies. |
| Vaccinium myrtillus | Benefits due to anthocyandin contents with particular antioxidant benefits on the eye, perhaps preventing eye complications of diabetes. |

| | |
|---|---|
| Korean Ginseng | May help energize and questionable effect on reducing blood sugar. |
| Opuntia ficus | Nopal is a Mexican botanical remedy for type 2 diabetes mellitus, but uncertain benefits may only be apparent with high dosage. |
| Ocimum sanctum | Holy basil has been reported to balance blood glucose and lower cholesterol in very limited studies. |
| Silybum marianum | The silymarin component of milk thistle is very versatile, offering liver protection, "detoxification", antioxidant effects and indications that it may improve blood sugar control, by unknown mechanisms. |
| Miscellaneous | There are many beneficial phytonutrients that can be advantageous in Syndrome X. These include antioxidants and specific botanical derivatives such as "natural" methyl inositol (pinitol) and flax seed meal which may work by its content of omega 3 fatty acid precursors. |

**Table 57**: Herbs and botanicals with potential benefits in the management of glucose intolerance, Type 2 diabetes and Syndrome X. These agents should be used with the advice of an expert healthcare giver. The safety, effectiveness and optimal dosage of these agents is not entirely clear.

## FUNCTIONAL FOODS

Hippocrates declaration in circa 400 BC was: "Let food be your medicine and medicine be your food". Physicians practiced this dictum for centuries, but with the pharmaceutical revolution its importance became relegated fifty years ago, only to re-emerge in this new millennium. These days, "functional food" (food that promotes health) has become a very important area of research and development in the nutritional (and medical) sciences.

The terms "functional food" imply that food can be selected, mixed or modified in a way that may prevent or treat disease, but regulatory authorities are cautious about disease treatment claims for food and new legislation is pending to define "medical foods". The US has been relatively slow to define "food as medicine" in comparison with several Asian countries, especially Japan. Functional food has created a new legal quagmire as disease treatment claims for food are highly regulated and the labeling of food versus dietary supplements is a hot topic. A dietary supplement when added to a food cannot automatically permit the food to carry a "health claim" of supporting body structure and function.

Against this confusing background, we can appreciate that functional foods may be very valuable in the combat against Syndrome X, especially given the availability of soy and beta glucan components of fiber for the creation of "functional X foods™". There are many areas of functional food development that are relevant to Syndrome X including new margarines, meat substitutes using soy and novel types of baked goods. Of all areas of food research, milk provides a good example of the move towards "functional beverages".

## Milk of Many Types

On the one hand dairy milk is touted for its nutritional benefits, whereas on the other it is constantly criticized for its content of saturated fat. Unmodified dairy milk presents a relatively high fat and cholesterol load, but it is a good source of calcium and vitamins. In recent years, the role of dairy milk components in the cause of allergies and immune disorders has been hotly debated and lactose containing milk is undesirable for many individuals who are intolerant to this principal milk sugar. These issues have led to attempts to modify dairy milk by additions or deletions or to the use of alternatives such as soy milk or ceveal-based milk e.g. oat milk.

The general consensus is that dairy milk can be quite healthful when used in moderation and modern processing has produced many types of milk which can be fitted to all needs. Fat free milk or skim milk is ideal for calorie-controlled diets but removing nutrients from milk tends to make it less palatable. To overcome these problems many new types of flavoring are available and "flavored milk" is very attractive to children. Whatever the perceived drawbacks of milk consumption may be, milk is a much healthier choice than soda or adulterated fruit juices that are often loaded with refined sugar (fructose). These circumstances make dairy milk an ideal basis for creating a "functional beverage", or a drink with special health benefits.

Dairy milk is notoriously difficult to work with in terms of flavoring or modification of its composition. Consumers tend to avoid "milk" that does not taste like whole milk. However, recent food research at Bravo Brands Foods Inc. (Palm Beach, Florida) has led to the development of modified milk that contain dispersible soluble fibers (beta glucans) that have multiple health benefits.

The use of miscible powders to add to milk for flavor or making a "milk shake" is very popular. Many of these powders are loaded with refined sugars and they are unhealthy. Bravo foods has a very important research initiative to create healthy milk additives (milk shake powders or "syrups") which can act as functional food and provide an appropriate alternative to unhealthy, existing flavoring powders or syrups. Reducing the fat content of milk reduces its pleasurable mouth feel, but this can be corrected by adding beta glucan components of oat soluble fiber which have good properties as a fat substitute. These new functional milks are very attractive to both children and adults. They provide the good basic nutritional content of milk with the versatile health benefits of beta glucans in a type of "smoothie" milk shake (The X-Smoothie™ Smoothie King Stores). Whilst soy milk and oat milk have some advantages for health they do not fit the Western palate. Dairy milk is a dietary staple in Western society and it has now come "full circle" as it forms a basis for health giving functional beverages.

## A COMBINED NUTRACEUTICAL APPROACH TO SYNDROME X

One may be impressed by the variety of remedies of natural origin which have a putative role in the combat against Syndrome X. Nutraceuticals that will impact insulin resistance in a significant manner are very valuable. The glucocolloid fraction of soluble oat fiber containing beta glucans forms a versatile substrate that is currently available to make dietary supplements and functional foods which may be beneficial in Syndrome X. The element chromium appears to play a very important role in the actions of insulin and mounting evidence indicates that it is a valuable natural approach. Whilst some concerns exist about chromium and DNA damage, such concerns are restricted to artificial circumstances of laboratory experiments in isolated tissues. The amounts of chromium given in these kinds of toxicity testing experiments far exceed levels that would be recommended for human consumption. Extensive clinical experience with chromium supplementation has not resulted in reports of common toxicity, even at relatively high doses.

A more indirect approach is the use of antioxidants with specific benefits in the prevention of the development of advanced glycation end products (AGES). These antioxidants include alpha-lipoic acid and carnosine. It is sugar and protein cross-linking (AGES) that account for many complications of diabetes mellitus and premature tissue aging. Soy protein and active forms of omega 3 fatty acids (notably, EPA) also prevail as beneficial in nutritional approaches to Syndrome X. The whole issue of elevations of blood homocysteine is not accounted for in many discussions of Syndrome X, but nutritional approaches to address this issue, with vitamin B6, B12 and folic acid, are seen as increasingly valuable.

Several dynamic and very valuable dietary supplements and functional foods have emerged with soluble fiber mixtures and the basic component of the beta-glucan extract of soluble fiber (US patent 6,060,519) to which can be variably added alpha-lipoic acid, chromium as picolinate or carnosine, carnosine alone and blood homocysteine reduction formulae. More innovative products are under development containing suitable forms of active omega 3 fatty acids (microencapsulated or powdered) and soy protein, or new forms of whole soy processing. I believe that these nutritional cocktails will form a solid, natural approach to combat Syndrome X and pilot clinical trials have produced exciting individual reports of welcome weight loss, substantial reductions in serum cholesterol and reductions in the need for medications directed at the treatment of the components of Syndrome X. Given the current lack of availability of versatile and safe pharmaceuticals to address more than individual components of Syndrome X, an integrated approach using behavioral medicine and nutritional principles is the most attractive first line option for the combat against Syndrome X.

## FUTURE SUPPLEMENT FORMULATIONS

Several dietary supplements have appeared with variable claims of benefit for controlling the components of Syndrome X. It is clear that soluble fibers from a variety of sources are potentially quite valuable for balancing blood glucose, reducing blood cholesterol, assisting with weight control and secondarily improving cardiovascular function. Oat soluble fiber and its extracts have good scientific precedent for their use in Syndrome X. There have been other important developments in the production of soluble fiber products that serve as ideal bulk ingredients for dietary supplements or functional foods. An interesting new fiber ingredient is maltodextrin which is produced from corn starch. This fiber is resistant to digestion, and like oat soluble fiber and its extracts, it is prebiotic in its actions and results in the production of short chain fatty acids in the colon. A variety of scientific studies, published in peer-review literature, show that maltodextrins can help maintain healthy intestinal function, exert favorable effects on glucose tolerance and reduce insulin response following mixed meals. Maltodextrins carry several patents, including one novel patent for food composition resulting in blood pressure-lowering effects. As the chemistry of soluble fiber becomes increasingly understood, several new extracts of soluble fiber will become available for the use in the combat against Syndrome X.

There is no doubt that the "sweet tooth" of Western society has caused health problems by encouraging excessive dietary intake of refined sugars. Increasing recognition of health problems, including Syndrome X, that result from the over-consumption of sugar has led many scientists to search for sugar substitutes. Such substitutes are preferred if they have taste characteristics similar to sucrose (table sugar) with the advantage of reduced caloric value and lack of any contribution to tooth decay. Commonly used alternatives to sugar have included, saccharin, cyclamates, aspartame, polyol sweeteners and botanical extracts, such as Stevia. Lactose (milk sugar) is often avoided because of the common occurrence of gastrointestinal intolerance to this sugar. Several alternative sweeteners have a poor taste profile which in some cases leaves a bitter after-taste in the mouth. Few artificial sweeteners have desirable textures or "mouth-feel" and polyol sweeteners may cause digestive upset. For example, sorbitol can cause diarrhea and excessive gas when taken in significant quantities. In contrast, there are sweeteners, produced by fermentation of corn starch (polyols), which have excellent digestive tolerance. Erythritol is a modified polyol sweetener which has been recognized as quite safe. Compared to other polyol sweeteners, erythritol is less likely to cause digestive upset. Some sugar substitutes are associated with claims of thermogenic properties and most alternative sweeteners have a low glycemic potential e.g., trutina dulcem.

Much has been written about the safety of sugar substitutes, including repeated concerns about side effects, long-term toxicity and even potential cancer promoting properties. Aspartame has been reported as a common cause of headaches and it may cause other neurological symptoms-effects that are denied by the manufacturers. Saccharin and cyclamates have shown significant toxicity in animals at very high dosage, as has the unapproved "sweetener" Stevia. In general, I believe that approved artificial sweeteners are quite safe and valuable for the dietary changes needed to impact Syndrome X.

## CHAPTER SUMMARY: AN ARRAY OF ESSENTIAL NUTRIENTS

Cardiovascular disease and Syndrome X cannot be shown clearly to be a dietary deficiency disease but lack of essential nutrients may play a role in its causation and progression. Increased intake of certain vitamins, minerals, essential fatty acids and soluble fiber, especially beta glucan forms of soluble dietary fiber have been shown to assist in blood cholesterol and triglyceride reduction. The omega-3 fatty acids that are found in fish oil (especially EPA) have a particular and favorable role in lowering blood lipids and they may help to increase insulin sensitivity. There are variable estimates of vitamin deficiencies in Western communities, but as much as 85% of the population may not have a consistent, optimal intake of vitamins, minerals, essential fatty acids or fiber. If an individual is not conscientious about his or her diet, the chance of deficiency of one or more essential nutrients is 100%! Calorie controlled diets may be lacking in essential nutrients and hyperglycemia causes excessive elimination of certain essential vitamins and minerals from the body.

Of considerable importance is the role of oxidation of fats in the genesis of atherosclerosis. It appears that oxidation of cholesterol and triglycerides is an important prerequisite and promoter of "fat" and cholesterol deposition in arteries. This oxidation can be prevented by nutrients that are antioxidants (notably vitamins C, E, beta carotene, selenium, zinc, phytonutrient antioxidants and many other antioxidant compounds). Certain antioxidants, e.g. carnosine and alpha lipoic acid, have potent and versatile actions in the combat against Syndrome X. The correct selection of food is important because oxidized fat is abundant in aged foods or meat, especially if they are poorly manufactured or stored. It seems clear that refined sugars plays a negative role in this oxidative process of fats, at least by interference with the actions of vitamin antioxidants.

There is a well-defined role for omega 3 types of essential fatty acids, soluble fiber or beta glucan extracts of soluble oat fiber, soy protein and antioxidants in the management of Syndrome X. These nutritionals exert effects on cardiovascular wellness dependent on or independent of a cholesterol-lowering ability. Soluble fiber or extracts of soluble fiber, soy protein and essential fatty acid supplementation of the diet are among the most important natural options that have emerged recently as prime candidates for dietary adjustments to promote cardiovascular health. They are versatile first line options to combat Syndrome X, Y and Z...

---

### Syndrome X: Nutritional Factors™

- **Soluble fiber**
- **Fish oil, EPA**
- **Vanadium**
- **Antioxidants**
- **Fermented barley products**
- **Selected herbs?**

- **Alpha lipoic acid**
- **Chromium**
- **Carnosine**
- **Soy fractions**

---

See www.naturesbenefit.com
and www.enzy.com

# SECTION 9

# SPECIAL AGES:
# SPECIAL CIRCUMSTANCES

### SOME ALARMING FACTS ABOUT CHILDREN

Despite the importance of lifestyle in the maintenance of health in both childhood and later life, there are relatively few accounts of "effective" methods to correct adverse lifestyle in children or adolescents. Attempts to analyze some of the health problems in the young reveals some alarming statistics on the health and well-being of children in North America. Table 58 summarizes some of these worrying observations of diet, lifestyle and physical fitness among American youth. A perusal of some of the statements on Table 58 are alarming and probably very revealing for many readers. These statistics are getting worse not better.

- Average duration of vigorous exercise, less than 15 minutes per day.
- Greater than 40% of calories from simple sugars, often.
- More than one-quarter may have high blood pressure.
- One-third have elevated blood triglycerides.
- One-half of all children may have high blood cholesterol.
- Two-thirds eat too much salt.
- Three-quarters eat excessive fat in their diet.
- Sixty-seven percent of all children have three or more risk factors for cardiovascular disease.

- All most 100% of all children have at least one major risk factor.
- Sixty-four percent of all children may fail to meet minimum physical fitness criteria.

**Table 58:** Some facts on levels of fitness, lifestyle and general health issues among children in the United States, based upon data presented by Dr. Charles Kuntzleman in his book entitled "Healthy Kids for Life" (1988).

## Scary Statistics

We can recognize Syndrome X as a part of a huge health problem that affects Western society. It is increasing in its occurrence in young children who are developing maturity onset diabetes of the young (MODY). The child with MODY often becomes an adult with full blown cardiovascular risks which may result in early death and disability. It is clear that 70 million Americans have Syndrome X in one form or another and this is mirrored by the known presence of about 61 million Americans who have cardiovascular disease. Adding components of Syndrome X to these numbers on an individual basis produces some shocking statistics. The combined occurrence of high blood cholesterol and or obesity with cardiovascular disease is estimated by some to affect about 160 million North Americans!

It is easy to see why lowering blood cholesterol has become a national obsession. Cardiovascular disease causes at least one million deaths per year and every twelve months more than 7 million heart attacks occur, with reports of about 5 million strokes. Cardiovascular disease "swamps" all other causes of death in the US.

## Surveys are Revealing

The support for strong statements on the poor health of our nations' children comes, in part, from the National Health and Nutrition Examination Survey (HANES). The HANES has implied that there is a direct relationship between the weight of a child and the amount of time that a child may spend watching television (or plonked at a computer terminal or play station). It has been estimated and data from the HANES implies that the occurrence of childhood obesity increases by approximately 2% for each additional one hour per week that a child watches television. Switching off TV (video games and computers) more often may be a very important, simple, public health intervention. The "couch-potato-phenomenon" appears to operate in adults to the same degree that it operates in children. The sad situation is that children tend to take their lead from adults. Sitting on a couch and sharing cigarette smoke, eating simple sugars, excessive salt and fat are obvious examples of Syndrome X-forming behavior.

## X–KIDS

Syndrome X is rearing its ugly head among US youngsters, but its level of occurrence has not been estimated with any precision. Researchers have stressed that cardiovascular disease due to atheroma germinates in childhood, whilst pediatricians have commented on the dangers of childhood hypercholesterolemia (high blood cholesterol) for more than forty years, in the presence of residual complacency. Dr. William Kannel of Boston University has coined the termed "atherogenic way of life" among young people and he has indicated that the average American child has a one chance in three of experiencing a cardiovascular catastrophe before reaching 60 years of age. Dr. Kannel has called for an expansion of the pediatrician's responsibility for health beyond adolescence.

The best-selling author Robert E. Kowalski MD has defined the importance of high blood cholesterol and other factors (obesity and sedentary lifestyle) in childhood, as it pertains to the occurrence of heart disease later in life. In his book entitled "Cholesterol and Children", (Harper and Row, NY, NY, 1988), Dr. Kowalski describes a combination of positive lifestyle change and nutritional interventions for dealing with cardiovascular risk factors. He stresses the problems of conventional treatments for childhood obesity, high blood cholesterol and diabetes, particularly in relationship to the use of pharmaceuticals. Dr. Kowalski makes a specific case for the use of soluble portions of oat bran for cardiovascular health in children – a matter discussed in detail in Section 7 of this book.

More than 50% of all children have at least one risk factor for heart disease and it is known from recent studies (Third National Health and Nutrition Examination Survey, Jan, 2002) that at least 6.7% of all young adults age 20 – 29 years have Syndrome X. It is known that up to one in five new patients attending pediatric treatment facilities in hospitals may have Type 2 diabetes and in the late 1990's local childrens' clinics in Southern California reported a ten-fold increase in the number of cases of maturity onset diabetes of the young (MODY) over a five year period. My best guess is that about 2% of all children may have Syndrome X and an unknown proportion of these kids may be less than ten years of age.

## EXAMINING ASPECTS OF POPULAR
## CHILDHOOD DIETS AND LIFESTYLE

Children are eating "piles of junk". It is recognized that most of American children (almost 100% !) will eat sweet deserts on at least six occasions in a week and that they may on an average drink about 24 ounces of soda per day. It is commonplace for meals to be taken outside the home, usually at fast food restaurants, and the occurrence of diets with inadequate levels of fiber and essential nutrients is often the norm. Many children are relative strangers to vegetable protein and essential fatty acids of the omega 3 series.

Exercise has been shown to be a key initiative for promoting health in childhood. I recommend this approach strongly and I am astounded at reports that only about one-third of all American school children receive daily physical education classes, which are often lacking in more rigorous forms of exercise. The Government has appealed finally for more attention to be paid to promoting lifestyle change among children in the US.

## CHILDHOOD NUTRITION AND CARDIOVASCULAR RISK

Contrary to popular belief, children and adolescents are not immune to heart disease. The acceptance of old notion that children are resilient to consequences of poorly planned diets and any food "that passes their lips is good for building their body" is one of the biggest mistakes ever made by the modern mother or father. Atheroma has its roots in childhood and evidence suggests that the children of modern times are accumulating an unprecedented burden of cardiovascular risk factors by engaging in lifestyle that will tend to result in Syndrome X. The media seems to avoid too much coverage of this mounting problem, perhaps for predictable reasons.

In terms of overall public health significance, education of children about healthy eating should be given priority. We are reminded often that coronary heart disease is the number one killer in Western Society and it starts in childhood. High blood cholesterol and hypertension is much more common in children than had been presupposed by many, including some members of the medical profession. America has the most obese youngsters in the world per capita and the increasing occurrence of diabetes (MODY) in childhood is frightening. It is not in anyway controversial to state that the dietary habits of the average child is often focused on fast-food items. Burgers and fries, or "fried anything", are often loaded with cholesterol, saturated fats and damaged unsaturated fats (trans fatty acids). When taken in continuity and excess, many types of fast or junk food are guaranteed to "break the heart".

## INTERVENTIONS FOR CHILDHOOD CARDIOVASCULAR RISKS AND SYNDROME X PREVENTION

How does one tackle this overlooked problem of childhood? The interventional principles to control cardiovascular risks in children are simple. Ideally, children should not be allowed to develop "bad habits". For a parent to let a child become permissively fat has been labeled by some to be a form of abuse. This type of rhetoric must be dismissed as counterproductive, but it helps define an increasing need for parental control. Childhood obesity in the US is tragically common, often impossible to reverse completely and it sets the stage for adult obesity. Whilst the causes of childhood obesity remain underexplored, several factors are known to contribute. Beyond some known genetic predispositions to obesity in children are the recognized contribution of emotional factors, family eating habits (or behavior) and misguided attitudes to food.

Children are receptive to positive attitudes about healthy food choices and their implications for weight control, athletic performance and "feeling good". Parents can do much to reinforce these attitudes and help "counter" the fast-food culture that has "consumed" Western society. To deny a youngster a visit to the eating parlor of their choice, once in a while, is probably wrong. It is the saturated fat, refined sugar and salt content of fast food that leads to the need to limit its intake. I am respectful of the fast food industry's (and general food industry) constant desire to examine and change the nutritional value of their meals to more beneficial compositions. After all, the fast food industry is fulfilling a consumer "need" which promotes the spread of "nutritional colonialism". Whilst I do not wish to deny anyone unhealthy types of fast food, its intake should be limited. Fast food parlours tempt even the most self-disciplined individual. Moderation is desirable. Like the alcohol abuser who may seek controlled drinking behavior, the time to instill controlled-eating-behavior is in childhood.

My indulgence in continuing to remind parents (including myself) about the obvious may not be perceived as constructive by some. However, the unfortunate issue is that many of our children have "established" nutritional problems. These nutritional problems are true examples of "malnutrition" that occurs often as a consequence of dietary excesses. Hypercholesterolemia and abnormal blood lipid profiles should be taken more seriously in childhood, at least when children reach school age. Dietary interventions in children often fail and drug therapy with lipid lowering drugs has to be avoided in childhood for safety reasons. Indeed, many lipid lowering drugs are contraindicated in most circumstances in children. Furthermore, the safety of anti-diabetic drugs in children has not been defined, but it must be now, given the alarming rise in MODY. Problems with drug treatments make natural nutritional interventions very attractive for use in children.

## DIETARY SUPPLEMENTS PRESENT OPTIONS IN CHILDHOOD: SOLUBLE FIBER AND SOY PROTEIN

One solution to the problem of established high blood cholesterol in children is the use of safe dietary supplements with blood-lipid-lowering properties. Clearly, soluble fiber, especially beta glucan extracts of soluble oat fiber can be used to lower cholesterol and balance glucose in children. Soy protein and soluble fiber extracts are to be preferred over drugs for lowering cholesterol in

children. The revered Italian physician, Dr. C. Sirtori, has emphasized the potential role of soy protein supplementation of the diet
as an effective means of lowering blood lipids in children. In fact,
Dr. Sirtori has gone as far as indicating soy protein inclusion in the
diet may be among first line options for lowering blood lipids in
childhood. I add soluble fiber and beta glucans from oats to this suggestion.

## BLOOD PRESSURE IN THE YOUNG

Adolescents and teenagers with hypertension (or obesity or
high blood cholesterol) are a difficult group to manage. Young
people are less likely to take notice of the serious nature of high
blood pressure as an important consideration in their day-to-day
activity. The profile of children with high blood pressure is often
recognizable, but not often spotted. Young people with high blood
pressure often have a family history of hypertension, they may be
obese and they may have a tendency to avoid physical activity. This
risk profile moves our children towards the components of
Syndrome X. Youngsters with these medical problems are not normal, but many US children or adolescents are beginning to match
the X-profile.

The acceptance of the status of the "chubby child" who will
grow out of their problem is a dangerous deception. Childhood
obesity is a sad reflection of our "advanced" society. Substance
abuse in teenagers must not be forgotten as an important underlying factor in the causation of elevated blood pressure. The healthcare giver or parent should be vigilant to spot drug abuse (e.g.
"drug speed" or "herbal speed", e.g. ephedra) and help the young
person correct this type of adverse lifestyle.

## BLOOD PRESSURE IN THE ELDERLY

Mature and elderly individuals are the commonest group in
which blood pressure lowering strategies are undertaken. It is recognized that the health risks associated with hypertension increase
as an individual gets older. The famous British Physician, Lord
Platt, described hypertension as a function of age. Whilst this was
a valuable observation, it caused some complacency about the treat-

ment of hypertension in the elderly. The mature individual must accept the concept that intervention for hypertension in the presence of advanced age is still very beneficial. Recent clinical trials have shown measurable benefits resulting from the reduction of both systolic and diastolic blood pressures in people over the age of 65, certainly to levels below 180 mmHg systolic and 90 mmHg diastolic (and lower).

Contrary to popular belief, the elderly may be a group for whom natural options may be an ideal treatment approach. I believe that elderly people with mild hypertension should always be considered a prime target for natural options or lifestyle intervention, rather than drug therapy. The reasons for this are obvious. Elderly people may not tolerate the side effects of anti-hypertensive medication and the benefits of "strict" blood pressure control in the elderly are still not as well defined as they are in younger people (see Section 4, Combat Hypertension). However, carefully conducted clinical studies have shown in fairly long follow-up periods of five years or more, that mature individuals can substantially reduce their risk of heart attack, stroke and renal failure by appropriate management of high blood pressure.

Specific factors are important in the treatment of an elderly individual with blood pressure, such that treatment interventions are only to be deemed appropriate when these factors are carefully considered. The aging process results in a situation where reflexes in the body are diminished in elderly individuals. Even in the absence of high blood pressure or the taking of anti-hypertensive medications, an elderly subject may become faint when they move quickly from a lying or sitting posture to the upright posture. This phenomenon of "orthostatic hypotension" is quite common in the elderly and, of course, it is sometimes made worse by the prescription of drugs that lower blood pressure.

Elderly people may be less attentive to their diet and may engage in frequent variations in salt or alcohol intake in their diet. Syndrome X is characterized by a hightened sensitivity to salt intake, causing hypertension. Substance abuse in the elderly is much more common than has been previously recognized by many healthcare givers. Self reliance (or plain stubborn behavior) may increase with age and elderly people may be very resistant to discussion about their lifestyle habits. Advanced age may bring to some individuals a tendency for relaxed behavior and errors of judgment. Measures that improve compliance with medication in the elderly are particularly important issue and it is recognized that errors in the taking of medication are quite common in the elderly.

Periodically, family members or healthcare givers should ask an elderly patient who is taking medications to empty their cupboard and present the contents for examination. It is quite surprising what elderly people may take in terms of over-the-counter remedies (dietary supplements and drugs). It is even more surprising these days that people will mix dietary supplements and prescription medications without any knowledge or concern or consideration for their potential interactions. These problems are not confined to the elderly, even though they may be more common in individuals of advanced years.

Finally, and very important, the human body has a decreasing capacity to handle both synthetic and natural medications with age and, therefore, adjustments of dosages of some medications or dietary supplements are frequently required in the elderly. Diminished kidney function occurs with age and this means that compounds cannot be excreted or metabolized by the body in a normal manner. Specific concerns for health maintenance in the elderly are of increasing significance as the elderly population increases and Syndrome X evolves. Whilst I have elected to discuss blood pressure control in the elderly, the same issues are relevant to drug treatments for lowering cholesterol and blood sugar in this age group. There is no doubt that the control of blood sugar with potent antidiabetic medicine and the use of cholesterol-lowering drugs must be carefully supervised in the elderly.

## Diet in the Mature Female

A woman seeking relief from menopausal symptoms is one of the commonest problems that faces a healthcare giver in Western Society. Many women, however, suffer in silence or they take the plunge towards synthetic hormone replacement therapy (HRT). Whilst the untoward symptoms of the climacteric (change of life) are troublesome, the post-menopausal onslaught of degenerative diseases, such as cardiovascular disease, is the real health problem that faces the mature female. New information has surfaced about the dangers of conventional HRT, which is provided in a synthetic format or in preparations derived from horses urine. Recent warnings of a three-fold risk of thrombotic episodes in women on conventional HRT has been "brushed under the carpet", as has emerging evidence that estrogen may not afford reliable protection against heart disease in the post-menopausal female. Estrogen replacement therapy may commonly cause weight gain and increased blood clotting tendencies which may contribute to the progression of Syndrome X. I am beginning to think that the perimenopause may be a trigger to Syndrome X in some women.

## DOES ESTROGEN REPLACEMENT THERAPY PREVENT HEART DISEASE?

Recent research shows that the relationship between estrogen and the prevention of heart disease in women is less clear than previously assumed. Researchers have reported recently that taking estrogen alone or in combination with progestins (progesterone-like drugs) had no beneficial effect on the presence of atherosclerosis of the coronary arteries of mature females. These findings further question the alleged benefits of estrogen replacement therapy which has been assumed to prevent heart disease and osteoporosis. These findings are predictable when one reflects on the "bouquet of barbed wire" of cardiovascular risk factors which must be impacted together to reduce the occurrence of heart disease.

## SOLUBLE FIBER AND SOY FOR CARDIOVASCULAR DISEASE PREVENTION

Soluble fiber or beta glucans from soluble oat fiber and soy protein containing modest amounts of isoflavones (approximately 2 mg/g) both lower total cholesterol with a corresponding beneficial change in overall blood lipid profile. The evidence for the promotion of cardiovascular wellness by soy protein supplementation of the diet has been well documented in animal and human studies which show not only lowering of blood lipids, but beneficial effects on other cardiovascular parameters, such as blood pressure and platelet function. The most relevant studies of soy in the promotion of cardiovascular health in the post-menopausal female are those that directly examine the effect of soy diets on post menopausal females. Ground-breaking research has demonstrated beneficial cardiovascular effects of soy protein and isoflavones. It appears that the cardiovascular benefits of soy isoflavones can also work in a manner that is independent of reductions in blood cholesterol.

Recent studies of post-menopausal females receiving soy protein containing variable amounts of isoflavones have shown positive influences on blood lipids and blood pressure. Soy may decreases the risk of cardiovascular disease in the post-menopausal state. Isoflavones in soybeans exert other cardiovascular benefits, including antioxidant properties which protect against low density lipoprotein oxidation and inhibition of platelet aggregation, resulting in an anti-thrombotic effect (anticlotting actions). The anti-thrombotic effects of isoflavones contrast with the thrombotic potential of conventional HRT. As an added bonus, soy isoflavones are weak estrogens that can control the symptoms of menopause (e.g. hot flashes).

## Many Benefits of Soy in the Post–Menopausal State

Soy protein containing isoflavones has chemoprotective effects against breast and colon cancer and the amino acid content of soy protein promotes renal health and calcium retention. The prevention and potential treatment of prostatic cancer by soy isoflavones, should catch the eye of those interested in the andropause of the mature male. A major component of the female menopause and male andropause is often Syndrome X. Several researchers have reviewed the laboratory and human evidence for the cancer protective effects of soy. Much evidence seems to link this cancer protective action of soy with the isoflavone content of soybeans.

A host of other studies suggest even more diverse health benefits of soy incorporation in the diet, including observations that soy protein isolates are good protein sources in weight reduction diets. Furthermore, genistein (a principal soy isoflavone) is antiangiogenic (interferes with unwanted new blood vessel growth in tissues) and it may play a role in the prevention or therapy of angiogenesis-dependent-diseases such as cancer, psoriasis, arthritis, and ocular disease. Proliferation of blood vessels in the retina of the eye occurs in diabetes and the antiangiogenic effects of isoflavones may be quite valuable in this situation.

Stephen Holt

## Elimination of Cardiovascular Disease and Longevity

The average person in Western communities may anticipate that they can live into their seventh decade. If coronary artery disease were able to be eradicated, about six years could be added to an individual's overall life expectancy. Approximately eleven years extra life could be achieved with the elimination of other diseases of the cardiovascular system, including stroke. This means that effective prevention of cardiovascular disease could result in an approximate average life expectancy for most people of approximately 90 years, versus the current average of 70 years. These projections reinforce the belief that a major enhancement of longevity will occur if we can combat Syndrome X. Effective combat against Syndrome X is one of the most important anti-aging tactics available to modern humankind.

Although aging results in declining cardiovascular function, there is evidence that good cardiovascular function can be maintained by a change of lifestyle and reduction of cardiovascular risk factors, even in some circumstances where such risk factors have been present for a considerable amount of time during early life. The idea that high blood pressure or elevated cholesterol should not be corrected in elderly people because it is "too late" is an outdated and inappropriate concept. It is never too late in engage in lifestyle modification to eliminate Syndrome X and promote cardiovascular wellness (see www.antiagingmethods.com).

## Syndrome X and the Premenopausal Female

In support of my concept of Syndrome X, Y and Z..., rests the major hormonal disturbances that can occur in premenopausal females in association with polycystic ovarian syndrome (PCOS). This disorder was reviewed in section 1 and it presents in its typical format with obesity, acne, irregular menstruation, excessive hair growth (male-type distribution) and infertility. The underlying change in body chemistry in this disorder involves insulin resistance which causes a switch in hormone secretions in the female body towards male-type hormones. This situation has justified the labeling of PCOS as Syndrome X of the ovaries, sometimes referred to as the Stein-Leventhal Syndrome. This condition is much more common than many appreciate and it occurs with a variable severity that is characteristic of the clinical presentation of Syndrome X itself. Some studies suggest that between 5 and 10% of all young women in the US may have some form of Syndrome X of the ovaries.

The cysts that affect the ovaries in PCOS may not cause any symptoms and they are not always detected by a standard vaginal examination. However, they are readily detected by pelvic ultrasound. Common reasons for an individual with PCOS to consult their physician include acne, obesity, excessive body hair, menstrual irregularities and infertility. The diagnosis of PCOS requires some degree of acumen because it is possible to have several of these common disorders in the absence of PCOS. The exact cause of PCOS remains unclear, but there appears to be a genetic tendency in some women where the sensitivity of the ovaries to the effects of insulin are increased. The treatment of PCOS is undergoing continuous revision, but evidence has emerged that lifestyle change with weight loss, exercise and tailored nutrition can be highly effective. Of course, this is the common approach to Syndrome X and PCOS is an example of how lifestyle can specifically affect reproductive health.

Although many of the symptoms and signs of PCOS improve with weight control and dietary change, open label observations imply that the use of beta glucan supplements, soy protein and fish oil may be quite beneficial. Conventional medicine has relied on treatment with female sex hormones (birth control pills with low estrogen formulations) and insulin sensitizing drugs. Drugs that block the production of male sex hormones (androgen-blocking drugs, such as spironolactone or finasteride) have been used, but I believe that there is a special role for the use of phytoestrogens of natural origin, especially soy isoflavones or perhaps polyphenol — containing extracts of red clover. It should be noted that insulin sensitizing medications (e.g. pioglitazone and rosiglitazone) do not lower blood sugar in people who do not have hyperglycemia, but these drugs can cause liver problems, as can hormonal treatments. Menopause is a "cure" for the common manifestations of PCOS, but insulin resistance persists and other manifestations of Syndrome X, Y and Z... may occur.

## SYNDROME X IN PREGNANCY

Pregnancy causes complex changes in the metabolism of the body with a specific tendency to result in hyperglycemia. About three in every one hundred pregnant women may develop Gestational Diabetes Mellitus and the underlying cause appears to be insulin resistance. This situation has led to the description of diabetes in pregnancy as a form of Syndrome X in pregnancy. Pregnancy-related diabetes has negative effects on the fetus with alterations in growth and development, together with some adverse, long-term consequences for the child.

The causes of insulin resistance in pregnancy are not fully understood. There may be changes in insulin receptor function, alterations in the effects of insulin in the liver and other changes in the chemistry of body tissues. In simple terms, the high blood sugar present in the mother results in "over feeding" of the fetus who develops hyperinsulinism (high blood insulin levels). This can result in abnormal fetal development and glucose intolerance in the neonatal period, resulting in hyperglycemia or serious hypoglycemia with other changes (e.g. respiratory distress, polycythemia or excessive numbers of red blood cells, low blood calcium etc). In fact, Syndrome X of pregnancy can sometimes result in a "form" of distorted, short term "Syndrome X" in the baby which is not characterized by insulin resistance.

The treatment of Gestational Diabetes requires special supervision because of dangers to the fetus. Good control of blood sugar is required in this disorder and natural approaches such as the use of soluble fiber or beta glucan components of soluble oat fiber may be valuable to complement conventional medical care. The value of omega 3 fatty acid supplementation in pregnancy is under-explored given the multiple potential benefits of these essential fatty acids which include: improvements in maternal insulin sensitivity, provision of building blocks for the fetal brain and the potential prevention of post natal depression. However, some caution must be exercised with the balance of active omega 3 fatty acids (EPA and DHA) to avoid undesirable changes in prostaglandin production (eicosanoid status).

I stress that self-medication in Gestational Diabetes is not recommended given the need to carefully supervise fetal and maternal well-being. It is not commonly recognized that the negative effects of Gestational Diabetes are not confined to the mother and fetus, they have some long lasting effects on the adult life of the baby and, perhaps, even future generations.

## Syndrome X Is Shaped In the Womb?

Scientific studies suggest that coronary heart disease may have its roots in the environment of the growing fetus. Changes experienced by the embryo, in utero, appear to be important in determining the occurrence of heart disease in later life. There is much evidence to support the idea that coronary artery disease may be linked to impaired fetal growth, particularly in the presence of Gestational Diabetes (Syndrome X of Pregnancy).

Studies in England and Wales of adult death rates from coronary heart disease show a relationship with death rates among newborn infants (in the early years of the 20th century). More detailed population studies, using statistics collected by the Medical Research Council (UK), show relationships between small weight at birth or disproportionate size of babies and coronary heart disease in later life. Low birth weight has been associated with development of the "insulin resistance syndrome" in later life. In addition, some research indicates that a newborn with a short body length in relationship to head size may have long-term abnormalities of cholesterol metabolism and blood clotting (Syndrome X).

Much of the research in this uncharted area of medicine has been highlighted by Professor D J P Baker of the Medical Research Council in England. His work points to a new research focus in prevention of heart disease. I believe that the data are strong enough to send another strong message about good prenatal lifestyle in women to ensure optimal well-being of the infant (and the adult). Programmed changes that affect health occur very early in our development. These are "neglected" preventive strategies for cardiovascular disease and Syndrome X.

## Syndrome X and the Liver

Abnormalities in liver function have been detected in obese individuals, especially in the presence of glucose intolerance. Fatty deposition in the liver of obese people has been recognized for many years, but it is only in the past decade that this disorder has been well-characterized in the medical literature. Dr. J Ludwig and his colleagues from the Mayo Clinic described a condition called "non-alcoholic steatohepatitis" or NASH. The description of NASH led to the definition of a spectrum of disorders of the liver that are related to obesity and type 2 diabetes mellitus or essential components of Syndrome X, (Mayo Clinic Proc., 55, 434-8, 1980).

The cumbersome terms "non-alcoholic steatohepatitis" (NASH) were coined to define a disorder that had tissue changes in the liver, similar to liver inflammation (hepatitis) caused by excessive alcohol drinking, but NASH is unrelated to alcohol intake. This spectrum of liver disease, associated with insulin resistance and Syndrome X, has been labeled in many cases as an example of non-alcoholic fatty liver disease (NAFLD). This type of liver disease is strikingly common and it has been noted to be present (at autopsy) in about one quarter of people dying in car crashes. It is estimated that as many as one in four or five people (up to 25%) in the general population of the US may have NAFLD and one in fifty (up to 2%) may have NASH. How many people progress from NAFLD or NASH to cirrhosis of the liver is unknown.

The only recognized treatment for this type of liver disease (NAFLD) is weight control. Surgery for the correction of major forms of obesity may make NAFLD worse. If diabetes mellitus is present with a "fatty liver" (NAFLD), then good blood sugar control may be beneficial in treating NAFLD. I believe that insulin resistance plays a major role in the development of what I have called Syndrome X of the liver. Whilst not all people with NAFLD have Syndrome X, almost all are obese. I postulate that the effective management of NAFLD can be approached by dietary changes, use of beta glucans, soy protein, effective antioxidants (e.g. Vitamin E, alpha lipoic acid and carnitine) and omega 3 fatty acids. To support my assertion, some studies of children with NAFLD show improvements with Vitamin E administration and other antioxidants may be beneficial.

Conventional medicine proposes several options for NAFLD including, metformin (biguanide drug therapy), cholesterol lowering drugs (clofibrate and gemfibrizol) and ursodeoxycholic acid (UDCA), a drug similar to bile salts that is normally used to dissolve certain types of gallstones. For reasons that are not clear, relatively little concern has been expressed about the use of statin type drugs in NAFLD. I believe that statin type blood cholesterol lowering drugs may be quite dangerous in some forms of NAFLD, especially NASH. Hepatoprotective natural therapies are worthy of consideration in NAFLD (e.g. milk thistle), but I believe that a special role exists for probiotic therapy (feeding friendly bacteria). My latter suggestion is based on studies that show a putative role for endotoxin products of bacteria to contribute to the worsening of NAFLD. This worsening of NAFLD can occur after bypass bowel surgery for obesity, where bacterial overgrowth in the bowel is common and is thought to contribute to the liver complications, experienced after intestinal bypass surgery for obesity.

## ETHNIC VARIATIONS IN THE OCCURRENCE OF SYNDROME X

A large amount of scientific data shows a greater tendency to develop Syndrome X and type 2 diabetes mellitus in several ethnic groups including Pima or Papago Indians in Arizona, certain Micronesian populations in Nauru, specific groups of Asian Indians (Gujarati Muslims, Punjabis, Hindus), Hispanics in the US and African Americans. The risks of the development of type 2 diabetes are particularly high in Pima Indians (50%) and certain Micronesians (40%) compared with Hispanics (about 18%) and groups of African Americans (especially mature African American females, 15-20%). The factors that determine the high prevalence of diabetes mellitus and syndrome X in these ethnic groups are beginning to be understood. Identified factors include lifestyle characteristics, common occurrence of obesity and genetic tendencies.

## COMBAT SYNDROME X IS A KEY TO ANTI-AGING (DÉJÀ VU)

We have learned that the eradication of diseases which result in death or disability is best approached by preventive medicine. Whilst the earlier that prevention is practiced, the better the outcome, disease prevention strategies are valuable at all ages. The plans to combat Syndrome X proposed in this book will impact the occurrence of cardiovascular disease – American's number one cause of death.

Many mature readers of this book are looking for practical ways to improve their general health and avoid or reverse the consequences of Syndrome X (or X, Y and Z…). In this book, I have taken a somewhat dim view of premature use of potent allopathic medicines (drugs) with some purpose. We have tended to forget the simple issues of listening to our bodies and tending its needs. The analogy I shall use is the idle car sitting in a garage. Left alone and not driven a car will deteriorate and ultimately fail. The same thing happens to the idle body. One important difference exists between a car and a body, the car is inanimate whereas the body has a master regulator – the mind.

We use the hyphenated "mind-body" term to express the notion that our systems have a generalized reaction to even simple stimuli, such as exercising. Whereas exercising creates both mentally and physically beneficial results, lack of exercise or even simple and minimal mobility can have a devastating effect on the body. If an individual sits in a chair with no stimuli, he or she will gradually experience decreasing mental awareness and a deterioration of physical health. This is a clear example of "disuse syndrome," a term coined by Dr. Walter M. Bortz in 1982 (J.A.M.A., 248, 10, 1203-8, 1982). In this context, "disuse" means that the physical needs of the body are given inadequate attention, which in turn leads to poor health and premature death. Men and women of any age with cardiovascular disease, and the older person who is at risk of heart disease, may rapidly go downhill if they stop engaging in physical activity. A sedentary lifestyle produces several predictable consequences, including obesity, a decrease in psychological well-being, musculoskeletal disorders, and premature aging.

Social interaction is at least as important an issue as physical activity to overall well-being. Everyone requires mental stimulation to maintain a sharp mind, just as they require social contact to nourish their emotional health. Without physical and mental stimulation, depression and a decline in cognitive functioning may result. Above all, the mind minds the body and the body can mind the mind.

My reason for re-inserting this "mind-body" section is because I believe that lack of motivation, feeling defeated and tendencies to "give up" are among the most important causes of perceived ill health. In the words of one of my many mentor's "It's not what you've got, it's the way that you live with it". Activity seems to be a key anti-aging tactic that may do more than any focused medical intervention.

There are many causes of aging that are within the control of an individual who makes a commitment to engage in a positive lifestyle. Readers are referred to the excellent practical suggestions of Dr. William Evans PhD and Dr. Irwin H Rosenberg MD in their book "Biomarkers" (Simon and Schuster, NY, 1991).

## X–Pets?

I cannot help noticing overweight cats and dogs who appear to be "swelling" in number. I am an animal lover with a great interest in the holistic care of animals (Holt S, Bader D, Natures Benefit for Pets, Wellness Publishing, 2001, www.wellnesspublishing.com). I have discussed these trends of increasing obesity in pets with several colleagues who are veterinarians or animal scientists and they were intrigued about the possibility of a form of Syndrome X in some animals. However, it is unlikely that the same metabolic factors operate in dogs or cats (primary carnivors)as in humans but fat rabbits and primates may be at risk for a kind of Syndrome X?

## Chapter Summary

Syndrome X, Y and Z… is relevant to all age groups. Special needs occur at special ages. Preventing Syndrome X must involve lifestyle and nutritional interventions in children. Tendencies to devlelop Syndrome X are shaped in early life. The combat against Syndrome X must not be too focussed on one age group. Lifestyle medicine and "natural" options figure for use in the prevention or management of Syndrome X at every stage in life.

# COMBAT SYNDROME X: CARDINAL COMPONENTS WITH CARDINAL APPROACHES

## SYNDROME X IN PERSPECTIVE

The components of Syndrome X are the leading cause of cardiovascular disease which is the leading cause of death in the United States. This perspective reinforces the fact that Syndrome X is the most important public health initiative to be addressed in the new millennium. Table 59 demonstrates the issues of death and disability which must be better recognized and brought to the forefront of medical preventive strategies. This reasoning does not even take account of the added "Y and Z" components of Syndrome X or Syndrome X, Y and Z...

| Cause | Number of deaths in 1996 |
|---|---|
| Heart disease | 733,834 |
| Cancer | 544,278 |
| Stroke | 160,431 |
| Adverse drug reactions | 110,000 |
| Chronic airways disease | 106,146 |
| Accidents | 93,874 |
| Pneumonia/Influenza | 82,579 |

| Diabetes mellitus | 61,559 |
| HIV/AIDS | 32,655 |

**Table 59**: Leading causes of death in the US in 1996, data from US Centers for Disease Control. If heart disease, diabetes, stroke and a portion of adverse drug reactions are added together and it is assumed that factors within the constellation of Syndrome X underlie many of these deaths, it is apparent that Syndrome X is, by far, our number one public health initiative.

This book started by defining Syndrome X as a set of risk factors and/or predisposing disorders for cardiovascular disease. I have expanded the concept to "Syndrome X, Y and Z...", to take account of the association of the metabolic components of Syndrome X with chronic inflammatory disorders, premature aging, liver disease, cancer and endocrinological (hormonal) disturbances. The occasional suggestions from some physicians to stop using the term Syndrome X has been overcome by the usefulness of the unifying concepts within this novel, medical label. Other terms have been proposed to describe Syndrome X including the "Atherothrombogenic Syndrome", "Reaven's Syndrome", the "Metabolic Syndrome" and the "Metabolic Cardiovascular Risk Syndrome". These terms or definitions underlying the labels are too narrow in describing the unifying concepts of the potential causation of several chronic diseases. Labeling diseases becomes important when "terms" can improve diagnosis and intervention. The terms "Syndrome X, Y, Z..." provide the broadest description of the disordered metabolism and stress the needs for a multifaceted intervention to combat "Syndrome X" (Y and Z). That said, acceptance of the terms require a recognition of the links within the X, Y and Z... of the disorders – debate will ensue.

The pivotal disorder within Syndrome X is insulin resistance which is caused, in part, as a consequence of excessive refined sugar intake in genetically susceptible individuals in Western Society. It is believed that this resistance to insulin determines the progression of glucose intolerance (hyperglycemia and occasional hypoglycemia) into Syndrome X and Type 2 diabetes. As such, these disorders may be perceived as the same illness occurring on a continuum, without automatic progression. I propose a extension of this continuum in my label "Syndrome X, Y and Z...

## SELF–IDENTIFICATION AND SELF–MANAGEMENT OF SYNDROME X

In these days of escalating costs of healthcare, there is a move to find more cost-effective means of dealing with common disorders such as obesity, high blood cholesterol and maturity onset diabetes. Market surveys show that 13% of households that can be described as consumers of natural products, and 12% of all other households, are engaged in the active management of diabetes mellitus. This latter circumstance is reported to be relevant to the family members of about 20 million Americans, which we know may constitute only the "tip of the iceberg". Recent studies have examined the benefits and effectiveness of "self-management- education" for individuals with maturity onset diabetes.

Dr. SL Norris and his colleagues from the Centers for Disease Control and Prevention have reported that education to help individuals with Type 2 diabetes manage their illness leads to positive outcomes, at least in the short term. (Norris SL and colleagues, Diabetes Care, 561-87, 2001). This report examined 72 studies published between 1980 and 1999 where the role of education in the management of diabetes could be assessed. Improving knowledge about Type 2 diabetes led to better controls over blood sugar and dietary habits, but these findings were not unanimous in all reviewed studies. Similar studies are required in Syndrome X.

It is clear that education to improve disease prevention and outcome is valuable, but in the case of Type 2 diabetes mellitus many researchers have stressed the need for a comprehensive approach that addresses all aspects of the disease in question. Throughout this book, I have stressed this issue in relationship to Syndrome X, where the approach must be multifaceted and broad-based. Conventional medical advice for the management of Type 2 diabetes has tended to concentrate on compliance with medications and monitoring of blood glucose, often at the expense of addressing lifestyle and nutrition. Education will improve disease outcomes, if the advice is focused on "evidence-based" approaches.

The evidence for lifestyle and nutritional approaches to combat Syndrome X is unquestionable, even though residual doubt exists with certain herbal or botanical approaches. Economic and practical issues dictate the need for individuals to take a pivotal role in self-care and I believe strongly that the first line options of diet, exercise and lifestyle change should be applied intensively in many cases, before the application of the standard allopathic, medical approach. In general, pharmaceuticals are "back-up" plans.

## Diagnosing Syndrome X

I have discussed "full blown" Syndrome X with its cardinal components of hyperlipidemia (high blood LDL, low HDL, high triglycerides), obesity, high blood pressure linked by the underlying state of insulin resistance. The early definitions of Syndrome X stress insulin resistance as the prerequisite for diagnosis of the disorder. Whilst arguments still prevail about the identification of Syndrome X, I believe that if an individual with insulin resistance has one or more of the constellation of disorders described in Syndrome X, then they have the disorder.

With my expanded concept of Syndrome X to Syndrome X, Y and Z..., spotting the metabolic syndrome could be problematic. It is known that the principal factors of obesity, high blood fats (dyslipidemia) and high blood pressure are cardinal components, but given the demonstrated links with other diseases (Syndrome X, Y and Z...) then disorders such as polycystic ovary syndrome, non-alcoholic fatty liver disease (NAFLD), gestational diabetes and changes in eicosanoid status  enter the picture. This is why I have proposed a Syndrome X Clinical Index to encompass the broad manifestations of the metabolic derangements and the disorders that result from the pivotal factors of insulin resistance in the conundrum of Syndrome X (or X, Y and Z...).

## Approaching the Detection of Syndrome X: The Syndrome X Clinical Index

Syndrome X remains hidden in a large proportion of the population, perhaps because many of its manifestations are comprised of "non-specific" symptoms or signs. Periodic health examinations and screening procedures have increased the detection of diabetes, high blood cholesterol, and hypertension (the cardinal features of Syndrome X) but simple low cost, screening strategies are required to detect people at risk for or with Syndrome X. These strategies involve the development of screening questionnaires combined with key medical findings that can form an "index" for detection or diagnosis. I refer to the development of this diagnostic index as the "Syndrome X Clinical Index"

The value of screening instruments for public health problems has been well demonstrated over the past thirty years. Examples include screening for alcohol or drug abuse and the development of risk indices for cardiovascular disease. These diagnostic tactics are based on a combination of clinical features (symptoms or signs) or laboratory indicators (e.g. blood tests) of the disorder to be detected. Screening instruments, such as these, work on a principle that the greater the number of disease related symptoms or signs present in an individual, the more likely that the individual has the disease in question.

My colleagues and I have developed several screening instruments to detect alcohol or drug related problems and probe aspects of adverse lifestyle (Skinner HA, Holt S, Schuller R, Roy J, Israel Y. Annals of Internal Medicine 101(6): 847-51,1984, Skinner HA, Holt S, Sheu WJ, Israel Y. British Medical Journal 292(6537): 1703-8,1986, Holt S, Skinner HA, Israel Y. Canadian Medical Association Journal 124(10): 1279-94,1981). When developing these indices of disease detection there is a requirement to validate the diagnostic accuracy of the components of the questionnaires or clinical or laboratory indications of the disorder. In the case of Syndrome X, attempts have been made to construct questionnaires or lists of medical tests with diagnostic ability, but these approaches have not been validated for their accuracy in the detection of Syndrome X (see books by Reaven G. and colleagues, Syndrome X, Simon and Schuster, NY, 2000 and Challem J. and colleagues, Syndrome X, John Wiley and Sons Inc., NY, 2000).

Table 60 proposes a combined "Syndrome X Clinical Index" that could be used in clinical practice to detect the risk or likelihood of the presence of Syndrome X. This detection program is based on my interpretation of medical literature that describes strong associations of certain lifestyle issues, symptoms and signs or medical findings in people with Syndrome X, Y and Z....

## Symptoms

- Symptoms of glucose intolerance, thirst, frequent urination, mental clouding, etc.
- Symptoms of complications of diabetes, e.g. changes in eyesight, sensory loss, etc.
- Irregular menstruation, infertility related to polycystic ovaries.
- Lifestyle issues e.g. sedentary living, excess refined sugar intake, excess high-glycemic- index-type food intake, substance abuse.
- Genetic tendencies, strong family history of components of Syndrome X
- Gestational diabetes, diabetes in pregnancy.

## Signs

- Obesity, "pot-belly" or "apple shaped body contour". More than 15 pounds over-weight.
- Skin or ocular manifestations of high blood cholesterol eg xanthelasma (cholesterol deposits in skin).
- Non-specific signs of diminished immune function e.g. recurrent yeast infection.
- Poor pulses in peripheral circulation (arteriosclerosis)
- Clinical detection of cystic ovaries or signs of the Polycystic Ovary Syndrome (Stein-Leventhal Syndrome), obesity, acne, excess of body hair in young females etc.
- Eye disease, cataracts, changes in the retina.
- High blood pressure sustained at greater than 140/85 mmHg.
- Liver enlargement due to non-alcoholic fatty liver disease (NALFD or NASH)

## Laboratory Tests

- Fasting blood glucose greater than 110
- Blood glucose higher than 140, two hours after the start of standard glucose tolerance test.
- Fasting blood HDL cholesterol lower than 40
- Fasting blood triglyceride greater than 200
- High total blood cholesterol with raised LDL of "dense type" (> 200 mg/dl)
- High serum fibrinogen and excess plasminogen activator inhibitor-1 (PAI-1).
- Biochemical evidence of liver disease with serum AST to AAT ratio less than 1 and normal serum alkaline phosphatase
- Elevated levels of serum ferritin?
- Increased androgenic hormones in females
- Genetic Screening?

**Table 60:** The proposed components of a combined clinical index for the detection of Syndrome X. The diagnostic "ability" of the proposed questions or findings has not been defined in field research. Any of these findings may variably assist in the detection of Syndrome X and the greater the number of these indicators that are present the more likely that Syndrome X is present or may develop. In general, laboratory tests have a high sensitivity and specificity for diagnosis. AST and AAT refers to blood tests aspartate aminotransferase and alanine aminotransferase, respectively.

It is known that certain components of the combined clinical index for the detection of Syndrome X (Syndrome X Clinical Index) will have greater diagnostic ability than others. This diagnostic weighting of the components of the "Syndrome X Clinical Index" requires measurement in population research studies. In other words, certain questions or findings in the index will have greater sensitivity and specificity for the diagnosis of Syndrome X –i.e. they have greater powers of diagnostic discrimination; where sensitivity implies the number of positive respondents that are truly positive for the risk or for the diagnosis of Syndrome X, whereas specificity refers to the number of negative respondents that are truly negative for Syndrome X.

## RETHINKING CAUSES OF SYNDROME X

There has been a tendency to view syndrome X as an automatic progression of events resulting from insulin resistance. However, the perceived consequences of Syndrome X may themselves operate to a variable degree, in a variable order, to create the complex clinical conundrum of Syndrome X. The "chicken and egg" argument (which came first) is dialogue that must be kept open, if advances in understanding are to occur.

Obesity is associated with the development of insulin resistance and several mechanisms for this link have been proposed, including changes in intermediary metabolism and hormonal changes e.g. resistin and perhaps leptin. The changes in eicosanoid status that occur in some individuals with Syndrome X may be primary events that alter responses to insulin e.g. alteration of the regulation of genes that affect insulins' actions by EPA.

Many factors alter insulin receptor number and function and the development of maturity onset diabetes mellitus involves a defect in the function of the beta cells of the Islets of Langerhans, in addition to any consequences of insulin resistance per se. There is a danger of "hanging one's hat" on insulin resistance as a final common pathway in the development of Syndrome X. Other factors operate.

From this line of reasoning at least two issues emerge. The first relates to an important broadening of the concept of Syndrome X to Syndrome X, Y and Z..., to create a more inclusive definition of the "hotch potch" of interlinked disorders. The second is that the combat against Syndrome X (or X, Y and Z...) must be versatile and it involves the unknown, given our incomplete knowledge of the clinical conundrum of Syndrome X.

## MISLEADING APPROACHES: FAILED TECHNOFIXES

It is human nature to err and even more "natural" to look for an easy way out, especially when addressing health issues. The preposterous claims of major weight loss "over a weekend", reversal of heart disease risk in a few weeks or short-term cholesterol cures are attractive, even to the logically minded. We have been the beneficiaries of quick fix reductions in the symptoms of disease with drugs, but we have not often experienced the pharmaceutical prevention or cure of common disease. This has led to our false sense of security that a "technofix" exists that will solve the health consequences of misdirected lifestyles.

"The quick fix" approach still dominates all forms of modern medicine and it is most readily identified in several alternative medical approaches. Many natural (or perceived alternative) approaches to disease prevention or management take a significant period of time to work. For example, taking a natural agent to lower blood cholesterol (or even a drug) may take many weeks before an optimal benefit is achieved. One of the biggest mistakes in the application of remedies of natural origin is to expect immediate or very short-term benefits. This mistake may lead to premature rejection of the natural approach on the grounds of its ineffectiveness. The reverse may apply to drug treatments where symptoms often improve in the short-term, but the disease that caused the symptoms persists because the drugs do not often access the root of the problem. Thus, predictable disenchantment can occur with any form of medicine if immediate gratification is expected. Chronic diseases evolve over extended periods of time and it is rational to conclude that improvements may take time, especially in the case of nutritional or lifestyle interventions. There is no "quick fix" for Syndrome X, Y and Z....

## READING LABELS: TRUE OR FALSE?

The US Government has attempted to protect consumers by demanding controls over the labeling of many products, especially food, dietary supplements and pharmaceuticals. There is an appropriate preoccupation with truth in labeling but even "truthful" labels can be misunderstood. The application of labeling in functional foods or supplements for Syndrome X provides a good example of potential consumer misunderstandings.

At first sight the need to restrict refined sugars in Syndrome X could lead us to choose products with low carbohydrate contents. However, not all carbohydrates are refined sugars. Soluble fiber is a carbohydrate of complex nature, but it is recommended for Syndrome X. Again the need for consumer education surfaces as paramount for the making of informed decisions on food or supplement selection. One may see why catch phrases such as "the low carb lifestyle" are misleading.

That said, there are problems with "truth in labeling". Some labels are "qualified" truths e.g. substantially free of genetically engineered food. This means that the food is not free of genetically engineered food (it contains a small amount!), e.g. soy, corn products, etc. Recent media attention has focused on labeling in common food or supplement items, especially meal replacement bars. It was found that a significant proportion of these bars have misleading labels with label statements not matching the contents of the product. In a national TV broadcast (Feb. 2, 2002) of a study by Consumer Labs, Inc., the notable proponents of the low carb lifestyle in the "Atkins' bar" were found to be particularly at fault by promoting a "low carb lifestyle" with a bar with significant carbohydrate content! The prevailing notion must be "caveat empeator".

## UNKNOWN CELLULAR DEFECTS IN SYNDROME X

Syndrome X and Type 2 diabetes are best viewed as a heterogeneous group of disorders with multiple causes. Whilst the disturbance in body metabolism that occur in the individual with Type 2 diabetes are well charted, the cellular defects that cause this disorder are underexplored. The metabolic defects or changes in the premonitory phases of maturity onset diabetes include a demonstrable resistance to the actions of insulin with compensatory hyperinsulinemia, followed by insulin lack, that can be demonstrated to be due to a defect in insulin secretion by the beta cell of the pancreatic endocrine mass. In association with these events are increased hepatic production of glucose with abnormal lipid synthesis and accumulation. The order of occurrence of these metabolic events is arguable and many metabolic changes are often linked to obesity and sedentary dispositions.

A fascinating hypothesis that links the metabolic changes in the progression of Type 2 diabetes or Syndrome X is the dysregulation of what has been termed the "metabolic master switch" by Dr. W. W. Winder and Dr. D. G. Hardie or "the fuel guage of the mammalian cells" (Hardie D. G. and Carling D, Eur. J. Biochem, 246, 259-273, 1997). This "metabolic master switch" is Adenosine 5 – monophosphate – activated protein kinase (AMPK) which plays a major role as a signaling system in regulating fat and carbohydrate metabolism and insulin secretion. AMPK seems to work as a metabolic master switch which responds to alterations in cellular energy.

The demonstration of wide-ranging actions of AMPK on liver metabolism, skeletal muscle, adipose tissue and pancreatic endocrine cellular function has led to the hypothesis that a change in the cascade of events resulting from the actions of AMPK could result in the principal metabolic disorders encountered in Type 2 diabetes including abnormal blood lipids, resistance to the actions of insulin and a resistance to the development of ketosis. Several factors modify the actions of AMPK including genetic defects, diet, aging and alterations in levels of aerobic fitness due to lack of exercise. The role of AMPK in the conundrum of the development of Syndrome X and Type 2 diabetes requires and deserves much further research.

## Looking at Food: How to Eat?

Several important recommendations for dietary habits are summarized in Table 61. The average American diet contains too many calories, too much fat, especially in a saturated form and it is lacking generally in vegetables, fiber and essential fatty acids of the Omega 3 series. The lower prevalence of cardiovascular disease in some countries compared with the United States or Western Europe is generally explained by the following differences in diet: lower saturated fat intake, higher fiber intake, more dietary inclusion of complex carbohydrates, lower total calorie intake and perhaps a higher ingestion of omega 3 types of essential fatty acids and soy. These differences emerge in part from a comparison of Western versus Eastern Asian dietary habits.

Considerable evidence has emerged that a movement towards a more "vegetarian-type" of diet results in several health benefits. However, the exclusion of meat or dairy foods is not necessarily required and some good arguments exist for their limited inclusion in a healthy balanced diet. The move towards a vegetarian type of diet is perhaps becoming increasingly acceptable in the West and it confers several advantages for health promotion. At first sight, these proposals seem tenable, but I have been impressed by the increasing emergence of the "fat-mature-vegetarian" in the past decade or so. This circumstance is real but poorly documented. Unfortunately, there are some vegetarians who consume large amounts of fruit, potatoes and pasta. These food preferences result in a high intake of sugar and they will not allow the potential protective effects of a vegetarian lifestyle against Syndrome X to be realized. I believe that the fat, mature vegetarian has been encouraged somewhat (or misled) by the USDA Food Pyramid Guidelines, which tend to promote the dietary inclusion of refined carbohydrates, especially refined flour and pasta.

Diets containing large fractions of vegetables and fruit tend to involve the selection of more natural foods which are not usually a concentrated sources of calories (low calorie density) with the advantage of their Low Glycemic Index. Care must be exercised with sugary fruits. Vegetables and fruits are bulky and induce a sensation of fullness after meals (satiety), which can help to prevent overeating. Furthermore, vegetables often provide adequate protein, a rich source of essential fatty acids, abundant minerals and vitamins and they are devoid of saturated or hydrogenated, unsaturated fats. Aside from these nutrient qualities, some vegetables have special health giving fractions, including phytosterols, phytochemicals, unabsorbable carbohydrates and fiber (Sections 7 and 8).

Not only should an individual examine the foods that are eaten to promote health, there is much importance in "better" dietary habits. These "habits" are important to consider because they involve behavior modification. Behavior modification of eating "styles" is a very necessary component of revising dietary intakes. Table 61 summarizes general dietary guidelines to combat Syndrome X.

| Initiative | Some Reasons |
| --- | --- |
| Caloric Consciousness | Prevents Obesity;  Lowers Cholesterol |
| Avoid High Cholesterol Foods | Often High Calorie;  Lowers Cholesterol |
| Eat Only When Hungry | Behavior Modification; Key to Weight Control |
| Avoid High Sodium Content Foods | Raises Blood Pressure; Fluid Retention |
| Decrease Animal Protein | Associated with Cholesterol in Diet, Promotes Osteoporosis |
| Avoid Refined Sugar | Raises Triglycerides;  Stops Antioxidant Functions |
| Increase Fiber Intake | Normalizes Digestive Function; Lowers Cholesterol; Cancer Protective |
| Increase Fresh Fruit and Vegetable Intake | Good Micronutrient Sources; Health Giving Phytonutrients |
| Switch to Vegetable Protein (e.g. Soy) | Lowers Cholesterol (Soy); Associated with Lower Incidence of Chronic Disease |
| Look for 100% RDA of Vitamin and Minerals (Vitamin Supplements Convenient) | Supports essential Body Functions |

| Supplement Essential Fatty Acid Intake, Especially Omega 3 Series | Essential for Body Functions lowers Cholesterol, Suppresses Inflammation |
|---|---|
| Read Food Labels | Avoid Undesirable Food Additives |

**Table 61:** Dietary Recommendations for combat against Syndrome X and the promotion of cardiovascular wellness. NOTE: Overall, a low saturated fat, low cholesterol, high fiber diet with adequate vitamins, minerals and important micronutrients is recommended.

Meals that are processed and "convenient" (usually as a result of "overprocessing") should be avoided when possible. Unfortunately, unhealthy food is often convenient and quite tasty. The health conscious individual should disqualify themselves from frequent visits to fast-food restaurants and try, whenever possible, to prepare their own meals from scratch. The act of preparation of food can lead to greater appreciation of food and sometimes diminished appetite. Snacking during meal preparation is best avoided, but for many this seems an impossibility. If snacking is desired, vegetables and fruit are the best option, not potato chips, or baked goods high in fat or trans-fatty acids and salt. I am a great proponent of the development of healthy snacks using functional food components with health benefits. If "snacking" is selected, let the "snacking" be healthy. There is no doubt that the act of preparing and taking well-balanced foods to the workplace is advisable, cost effective and "temptation" reducing.

There are some little tricks for better eating. Chewing food thoroughly may help suppress appetite and it improves the digestive process. Making more of a "ritual" of a meal is useful, with the setting of time aside and even the use of a stopwatch to lengthen eating time. The individual who eats to a sensation of fullness has usually overeaten. Some experts advise a departure from the dinner table with some residual hunger, but this is a difficult feat for many. Individuals who starve, have binges, vomit of their own volition, or have strange emotions about food, may have an eating disorder. For this situation, an experienced professional's advice is required!

Table 61 provides some simple guidelines to assist an individual in planning meals to prevent cardiovascular disease. It is generally accepted by most healthcare givers that less than 30% of the total calories in a diet should originate from fat but more healthy types of fat (up to 40% of total calories) are allowable in diets aimed at dealing with Syndrome X. The importance of the type of fat included in this 40% allowance must be clear. About 50-60 % of the total fat derived calories should be derived ideally from monounsaturated fats and polyunsaturated fats with a need to balance omega 3 and omega 6 fatty acid intake. The total daily intake of cholesterol should not exceed 300 mg and the incorporation of at least 30 grams of dietary fiber per day into the diet is ideal, preferably with the inclusion of beta glucan components of soluble fiber or extra soluble fiber, especially from oats or pectin or guar gum. More emphasis has been placed on limiting saturated fat intake, but it should be emphasized that when carbohydrate is substituted for saturated fat, as is so often the case, there is a risk of the body producing saturated fat from carbohydrates. This occurs "always" if calorie intake exceeds the body's requirements. The avoidance of refined sugars (carbohydrates) from foods with a high glycemic index is highly recommended. The importance of essential fatty acid inclusion (especially EPA and DHA from fish oil) in the diet to promote cardiovascular health should not be underestimated.

There are several sources of evidence that dietary and other lifestyle changes can stop the progression of coronary heart disease and reverse the process of atheroma in some cases. The benefit of lifestyle change in preventing or reversing heart disease or atheroma has become better defined. The idea that heart disease due to atheroma can be reversed by good lifestyle and nutrition has been around for about a long time, but it took 50 years of arguments to be registered as a credible current treatment approach.

## THE MISSING LINKS ARE DISCOVERED?

The majority of the general public may believe that a measure of health may exist in many of the popularized dietary approaches, including but not limited to the approaches of Atkins, Stillman, Ornish, Pritikin, Sears and others. Only Dr. Dean Ornish has presented clear evidence of benefit that a movement of the diet towards vegetarian habits with strict lifestyle change is both safe and effective in promoting health. It is reasonable to state that comparisons among diets may be unfair to a certain degree because they are "apples" and "oranges". For example, Atkins conceived his plans primarily with weight loss in mind and Pritikin had cardiovascular health at the root of this thoughts. Sears had a mythical health "Zone" in mind. Despite good intentions, modern science shows that specific approaches are not portable and diets need "tailoring". The objective of dietary approaches must include a general health initiative and these diets often fail in this regard.

Many modern nutritionists have endorsed the nutritional benefit of vegetable protein and dismissed the notion that animal protein is nutritionally "superior" to vegetable protein. If calorie intake is even only moderate with a balanced diet, there is no risk of amino acid or protein deficiency. The myth of the risk of protein deficiency during average dieting regimens should be dispelled. Several studies have indicated that there is as much of a relationship (correlation) between excessive animal protein intake in the diet and mortality (death) from coronary heart disease, as there is between dietary saturated fat intake and heart disease. Of course, animal protein often brings with it a high saturated fat content and a cholesterol burden, but excessive amounts of animal protein in diets may, per se, exert negative health effects. Furthermore, recent evidence shows abnormal protein metabolism in type 2 diabetes mellitus and, by inference, in Syndrome X. The negative health effects of animal protein- rich diets appear to operate in a manner independent of their saturated fat or cholesterol content.

## SOY, ESSENTIAL FATTY ACIDS AND FIBER PREVAIL

The emerging keys to healthy cardiovascular health and weight control approaches by diet are found in a move towards enhanced intake of plant protein, omega 3 fatty acid supplementation and enhanced dietary incorporation of fiber (especially beta glucan fractions of soluble fiber). Although obvious to many, putting this "all together" is a relatively new concept in dietary approaches to weight control, general health and, in particular, cardiovascular health. However, chewing cardboard-like material (insoluble fiber), choking on tofu or retching on cod liver oil may not be acceptable to many, even though it could be perceived as necessary by some. The mechanism of incorporation of these nutrients into the diet is very important. This is part of the basis of my recommendation for the appropriate use of palatable, inexpensive dietary supplements that can be readily incorporated into nutritional programs to promote health.

## PULLING IT ALL TOGETHER

I reiterate that unlike many books on natural health, this book has not been a series of pretty pictures, promises of exotic cures or recommendations for a "way-out" lifestyle. It is apparent that there are many natural ways to cardiovascular health and even more apparent that many of these ways to health may be based in simple common sense. The concepts of Syndrome X (or X, Y and Z...) provide a basis upon which lifestyle and nutritional changes can be applied.

The "bouquet of barbed wire" contains many damaging factors for cardiovascular health and these factors are not amenable to a single intervention. Some members of the dietary supplement industry who promise a beneficial outcome from a simple herbal intervention are as misguided as the physician who prematurely prescribes a synthetic medication for a lifestyle disorder. The pathway to combat Syndrome X (or Syndrome X, Y and Z...) is becoming increasingly clear, but it is complex and multifaceted in its approach. Table 62 represents a simple overview on "pulling it all together" to combat Syndrome X.

-      Education on syndrome X, with its extensions to Syndrome X, Y and Z..., is an absolute prerequisite.
-      Self-identification and intervention for adverse lifestyle is a cornerstone of successful management of Syndrome X.
-      Greater knowledge of the unifying concepts within Syndrome X may be required by healthcare givers, so that their management approaches may be multifaceted.
-      Screening for Syndrome X in clinical practice e.g. The Syndrome X Clinical Index (to be validated).
-      Focus on weight control, exercise, positive lifestyle change and changing behavior "together".

- Dietary interventions are among first line options. At present allopathic options fit "back up plans".
- Greater application of functional foods and dietary supplements.

**Table 62:** "Pulling it all together" in a simplified manner to Combat Syndrome X (X, Y and Z...).


CONCLUSION

Syndrome X, Y and Z... is a "can of worms" in which the worms have different identities and their relationships are linked by a common bond (or bonds). One aspect of this common bond is resistance to insulin. My hypotheses on the genesis of Syndrome X, Y and Z... have relied on the work of thousands of researchers and their efforts must be applauded and acknowledged. I trust that my "synthesis" of scientific fact and speculation has shed light on the most important health initiative of this millennium – our need to "Combat Syndrome X (or X, Y and Z...).

# AFTERWORD

The process of self-identification of a health problem with effective self-intervention (self-help) has been variably incorporated into society. This leads to improved public health and less dependence on visits to the doctors and pharmaceutical treatments. The extent to which an average person can provide self-help is only limited by education; and the power of self-doctoring has been shown in studies in England and Scandinavia. In these studies most people were found to initiate their own treatments correctly even prior to medical consultation. However, I am not suggesting that we do away with physicians or drugs or surgery, but self-help can do more to change the occurrence and clinical course of chronic disease than any hypothetical "technofix".

As the new millennium progresses, a more holistic health movement emerges and medical pluralism unfolds. Evidence exists that our society has an overdependence on drug therapies and between 35 and 45 % or more of all drugs may be prescribed for conditions for which they may not be indicated or totally effective. Nowhere are these circumstances more obvious than in the combat against Syndrome X and its sequelae. Whilst new drug developments may assist in the management of the constellation of disorders within Syndrome X, this disease conundrum is primarily related to lifestyle (a controllable variable) and genetics. Lifestyle disorders are best managed by lifestyle changes, not by drugs.

The terms "Syndrome X" have been used to describe the combination of obesity, hypertension and hypercholesterolemia, linked by underlying insulin resistance. Approximately 70 million Americans have Syndrome X which is causally linked with the development of cardiovascular disease (metabolic Syndrome X), female endocrine disorders, polycystic ovaries, non-alcoholic fatty liver disease, gestational diabetes, changes in eicosanoid status and cancer (Syndrome X, Y, and Z...). Syndrome X is caused by a combination of adverse lifestyle and genetic predispositions and it has variable clinical manifestations, which are apparent in the newly proposed "Syndrome X Clinical Index". Effective prevention and treatment of Syndrome X involves a multifaceted approach to impact all cardinal components of the disorder. Current allopathic treatments may have been too focused on individual components of Syndrome X and they tend to form a "back up plan" for management. In contrast, natural approaches with lifestyle modification and nutritional and/or nutraceutical interventions may provide versatile and powerful, first-line management options.

Evolution of research into soluble components of dietary fiber has led to the discovery of fractions of oat soluble fiber (beta glucans) which have been shown to effectively lower blood cholesterol, reduce post-prandial blood glucose and induce satiety and appetite suppression. Whilst these soluble fibers and especially beta glucan containing glucocolloids have physico-chemical properties that modulate gastrointestinal motility (delay gastric emptying) and retard or impede specific macronutrient absorption (glucose and fats), they have intrinsic metabolic effects (IMEF), largely as a consequence of their fermentation in the colon to produce short - chain fatty acids (proprionate, aceto-acetate and butyrate). Propionic acid can enter the portal circulation of the liver and interfere with cholesterol synthesis by blocking HMG CoA-reductase enzyme activity.

Recent research has underscored the importance of eicosanoid changes in Syndrome X and it is known that eicosapentanoic acid (EPA) can enhance insulin sensitivity by presumed effects on PPAR-receptors, which regulate the actions of insulin. These observations open up the pathway of the development of "genomenutraceuticals". Dietary approaches to weight control require reappraisal, as high saturated fat diets designed to induce dietary ketosis or diets involving protein-loading masquerade as the meritorious "low carb lifestyle". Diets to combat Syndrome X should have more liberal "healthy fat" recommendations (omega 3 and 6 fatty acids in the correct balance) with strict control of refined carbohydrate intake, restricted salt intake, enhanced fiber intake and a move toward vegetable sources of protein (e.g. soy foods).

The "balancing" effects of soluble fiber on blood glucose are part of the concept of the Glycemic Index of food, which is relevant to new dietary guidelines to combat Syndrome X. A major component of the "Glycemic Index" of food is related to altered rates of sugar absorption, determined to a significant degree by altered rates of transfer of glucose to its site of maximal absorption in the small bowel (a function of gastric emptying rate). Currently, Alternative and Complementary Medicine may have more to offer the prevention and treatment of Syndrome X than many existing pharmaceuticals, which are being scrutinized increasingly in terms of their cost effectiveness and safety. Combat against the components of Syndrome X, Y and Z... has become one of the most important current public health initiatives in Western Society.

---

**Combat Syndrome X**

1. **Public Education**
2. **Lifestyle Change**
3. **Nutritional Interventions**
   **(Syndrome X: nutritional factors™)**
4. **Current Allopathic Approaches**
   **form "back-up" plans**

see www.combatsyndromeX.com

---

# REFERENCES

## Author's comment

The author reviewed several hundred books and several thousand references or abstracts during the preparation of this book. Contained within books or journal articles listed below are other references relevant to the subject. The author has selected those references that form a pathway of potential research for an individual to seek further background and information. As such, the reference list provided below must be considered selective and references are categorized as A) Books of interest B) Articles of interest and C) Basic resources.

## Books of Interest

Annis E R, *Code Blue, Health Care in Crisis*, Regnery Gateway, Washington, DC, 1993.

Bernstein R K, *Dr. Bernstein's Diabetes Solution: A Complete Guide to Achieving Normal Blood Sugars*, Little Brown and Company, Boston, 2000.

Blaylock R, *Excitotoxins: The Taste That Kills*, Health Press, Santa Fe, 1994.

Broadhurst C L, *Diabetes: Prevention and Cure*, Kensington, NY, NY, 1999.

Challem J, Berkson B, Smith M D, *Syndrome X*, John Wiley & Sons, Inc., 2000.

Corea G, *The Hidden Malpractice*, William Morrow and Company, Inc., NY, NY, 1977.

Cowett R M, *Diabetes*, Raven Press, NY, NY, 1995.

Daneman D, Marcia F, Kusiel P, *When a Child Has Diabetes*, Firefly, NY, NY, 1999.

Dufty W, *Sugar Blues*, Warner Books, NY, NY, 1976.

Eades M R, Eades M D, *Protein Power*, Bantam Books, NY, NY, 1996.

Evans G, *Chromium Picolinate*, Avery Publishing Group, Garden

City Park, NY, 1996.

Evans W, Rosenberg I H, Thompson J, *Biomarkers, The 10 Determinantes of Aging You Can Control,* Simon & Schuster, NY, NY, 1991.

Fink D H, *Release From Nervous Tension,* Simon & Schuster Inc., NY, NY, 1962.

Gracey M, Kretchmer N, Rossi E, *Sugars in Nutrition,* Raven Press, NY, NY, 1991.

Greene B, Winfrey O, *Make The Connection, Ten Steps To A Better Body—And A Better Life,* Harpo Inc, NY, NY, 1996.

Gross M L, *The Psychological Society,* Random House, NY, NY, 1978.

Holt S, *Natural Ways to Digestive Health,* M. Evans and Company, Inc., NY, NY, 2000.

Holt S, *The Natural Way to a Healthy Heart,* M. Evans and Company Inc, NY, NY, 1999.

Holt S, *The Soy Revolution,* Dell Publishing, NY, NY, 1999.

Kowalski R E, *Cholesterol & Children,* Harper & Row, Publishers Inc., NY, NY, 1988.

Lafavore M, Editor, *Men's Health Today* (1998), Rodale Press, Inc., 1998.

Leeds A, Brand Miller J, Foster-Powell K, Colagiuri S, *The Glucose Revolution,* Hodder and Stoughton, London, UK, 1998.

Libov C, *Beat Your Risk Factors,* Plume, NY, NY, 1999.

McCool M H, Woodruff S, *My Doctor Says I Have A Little Diabetes,* Avery, Garden City Park, 1998.

Miller J B, Foster-Powell K, Colagiuri S, *The G.I. Factor,* Hodder Headline Australia PTY, Ltd., Rydalmere, Australia, 1996.

Norman JC (Editor), *Medicine In The Ghetto,* Meredith Corporation, NY, NY, 1969.

Pescatore F, *Feed Your Kids Well: How to Help Your Child Lose Weight and Get Healthy,* John Wiley and Sons, NY, NY, 2000.

Reaven G, Kristen Strom T, Fox B, *Syndrome X, Overcoming the Silent Killer that can give you a Heart Attack,* Simon & Schuster, NY, NY, 2000.

Romaine D S, Marks J B, *Syndrome X, Managing Insulin Resistance,* Harper Collins Publishers Inc., NY, NY, 2000.

Sale K, *Human Scale*, Coward McCann & Geoghegan, NY, 1980.

Sears B, Lawren B, Enter *The Zone, A Dietary Road Map*, Harper Collins Publishers Inc., NY, NY, 1995.

Sentochnik DE, Elipoulos GM, Infection and diabetes, In: Kahn CR, Weir GC, eds. *Joslin's Diabetes Mellitus*, Malvern, PA: Lea & Febiger, 1994:867.

Shadman AJ, Clark L, *Who Is Your Doctor and Why?*, Keats Publishing Inc., New Canaan, CT, 1980.

Simopoulos A P, Robinson J, *The Omega Plan*, Harper Collins, NY, NY, 1998.

Sosin AE, Sobell S, *The Doctor's Guide to Diabetes and Your Child*, Kensington Publishing Corp, NY, NY, 2000.

Steward HL, Bethea MC, Andrews SS, Balart LA, *Sugar Busters*, The Ballantine Publishing Group, 1998.

Stewart EW, The Troubled Land, Social Problems in Modern America, McGraw-Hill Inc., NY, NY, 1972.

Touchette N, *The Diabetes Problem Solver*, American Diabetes Association, Alexandria, VA, 1999.

Tuan YF, Topophilia, *A Study Of Environmental Perception, Attitudes, And Values*, Prentice-Hall Inc., Englewood Cliffs, NJ, 1974.

Weir GC, Leahy JL, Pathogenesis of non-insulin-dependent diabetes mellitus, In: Kahn CR, Weir GC, eds. *Joslin's Diabetes Mellitus*, ed 13, Philadelphia: Lea Febiger, 1994:240.

ARTICLES OF INTEREST

Anderson RA, Chen N, Bryden NA, et al., Elevated intakes of supplemental chromium improve glucose and insulin variables in individuals with type 2 diabetes, *Diabetes*, 46,1786-1791, 1997.

Anderson RE, Wadden TA, Bartlett SJ, et al., Effects of lifestyle activity vs, structured aerobic exercise in obese women, *JAMA*, 281,335-340, 1999.

Ascherin A, Willett WC, Health effects of trans fatty acids, *American Journal of Clinical Nutrition*, 66(suppl),1006S-1010S, 1997.

Austin MA, Breslow JL, Hennekens CH, Buring JE, Willett WS, and Krauss RM, Low-density lipoprotein subclass patterns and risk of myocardial infarction, *JAMA*, 260,1917-1921, 1988

Axelrod L, Kleinman K, et al., Effects of a small quantity of omega-3 fatty acids on cardiovascular risk factors in NIDDM, *Diabetes Care*, 17,37-44, 1994.

Baynces JW, Role of oxidative stress in development of complications in diabetes, *Diabetes*, 40,405, 1991.

Beck-Nielsen H, Hother-Nielsen O, Vaag A, Alford E, Pathogenesis of type 2 (non-insulin-dependent) diabetes mellitus: the role of skeletal muscle glucose uptake and hepatic glucose production in the development of hyperglycemia. A critical comment, *Diabetologia*, 37,217, 1994.

Cameron NE, Cotter MA, Horrobian DH, et al., Effects of alpha-lipoic acid on neurovascular function in diabetic rats: Interaction with essential fatty acids, *Diabetologia*, 41,390-399, 1998.

Carantoni M, Abbasi F, Warmerdam F, et al., Relationship between insulin resistance and partially oxidized LDL particles in healthy, nondiabetic volunteers, Arteriosclerosis, Thrombosis and Vascular Biology, 18,762-767, 1998.

Cariello A, Bortolotti N, Crescentini A, et al., Antioxidant defences are reduced during the oral glucose tolerance test in normal and noninsulin-dependent diabetic subjects, *European Journal of Clinical Investigation*, 28,329-333, 1998.

Cariello A, Bortolotti N, Pirisi M, et al, Total plasma antioxidant capacity predicts thrombosis-prone status in NIDDM patients, *Diabetes Care*, 20,1589-1593, 1997.

Castelli WP, Garrison RJ, Wilson PWF, Abbot RO, Kalonsadian S, and Kannel WB, Incidence of coronary heart disease and lipoprotein cholesterol levels: the Framingham Study, *JAMA*, 256,2835-2837, 1986.

Ceriello A, Bortolotti N, Motz E, et al., Meal-generated oxidative stress in type 2 diabetic patients, *Diabetes Care*, 21,1529-1533, 1998.

Chang RJ, Nakamura RM, Judd HI, Kaplan SA, Insulin resistance in non-obese patients with polycystic ovarian disease,

J. Clin. Endocrinol Metab., 57,356, 1983.

Cleland SJ, Petrie JR, Ueda S, et al., Insulin as a vascular hormone: Implications for the pathophysiology of cardiovascular disease, Clinical and Experimental Pharmacology and Physiology, 25,175-184, 1998.

Coulston A, Greenfield M, Kraemer F, Tobey T, and Reaven GM, Effects of source of dietary carbohydrate on plasma glucose and insulin responses to test meals in normal subjects, Am. J. Clin. Nutr., 33,1279-1282, 1980.

Coulston AM, Liu GC, Reaven GM, Plasma glucose, insulin and lipid responses to high-carbohydrate low-fat diets in normal humans, Metabolism, 32,52-56, 1983.

Czech M, The nature and regulation of the insulin receptor: structure and function, Annu. Rev. Physiol., 57,357, 1985.

DeFronzo RA, Ferrannini E, Insulin resistance: A multifaceted syndrome responsible for NIDDM, obesity, hypertension, dyslipidemia, and atherosclerotic cardiovascular disease, Diabetes Care, 14,173, 1991.

Durrans D, Taylor TV, Holt S, Intragastric device for weight loss. Effect on energy intake in dogs, Digestive Diseases and Sciences, 36(7), 893-6, 1991.

Exton JH, Hormonal control of gluconeogenesis, Adv. Exp. Med. Biol., 111,125, 1979.

Faccini F, Coulston AM, Reaven GM, Relation between dietary vitamin intake and resistance to insulin-mediated glucose disposal in healthy volunteers, American Journal of Clinical Nutrition, 63, 946-949, 1996.

Faccini FS, Hollenbeck CB, Jeppesen J, Chen Y-DI, and Reaven GM, Insulin resistance and cigarette smoking, Lancet, 339, 1128-1130, 1993.

Faccini FS, Riccardo A, Stoohs A, and Reaven GM, Enhanced sympathetic nervous system activity ñ the linchpin between insulin resistance, hyperinsulinemia, and heart rate, Am. J. Hypertens., 9, 1013-1017, 1996.

Fanaian M, Szilasi J, Storlien L, et al., The effect of modified fat diet on insulin resistance and metabolic parameters in type II diabetes, Diabetologia, 9, A7, 1996

Foster DW, From glycogen to ketones ñ and back, Diabetes, 33, 1188, 1984.

Farquahar, JW, Frank A, Gross RC and Reaven GM, Glucose, insulin and triglyceride responses to high and low carbohydrate diets in man, J. Clin. Invest., 45, 1648-1656, 1996.

Fuh MM-T, Shieh SM, Wu DA, Chen Y-DI, and Reaven GM, Abnormalities of carbohydrate and lipid metabolism in patients with hypertension, Arch. Int. Med., 147, 1035-1038, 1987.

Ginsberg H, Olefsky JM, and Reaven GM, Further evidence that insulin resistance exists in patients with chemical diabetes. Diabetes, 23, 674-678, 1974.

Ginsberg H, Olefsky JM, Kimmerling G, Crapo P, and Reaven GM, Induction of hypertriglyceridemia by a low-fat diet, J. Clin. Endocrinol. Metab., 42, 729-735, 1976.

Greene DA, Lattimer S, Ulbrecht J, Carroll P, Glucose-induced alterations in nerve metabolism: current perspective on the pathogenesis of diabetic neuropathy and future directions for research and therapy, Diabetes Care, 8, 290, 1986.

Hollenbeck C, and Reaven GM, Variations in insulin-stimulated glucose uptake in healthy individuals with normal glucose tolerance, J. Clin. Endocrinol. Metab., 64, 1169-1173, 1987.

Hollenbeck CB, Chen N, Chen Y-DL, and Reaven GM, Relationship between the plasma insulin response to oral glucose and insulin-stimulated glucose utilization in normal subjects, Diabetes, 33, 460-463, 1984.

Hollenbeck CB, Haskell W, Rosenthal M, and Reaven GM, Effect of habitual physical activity on regulation of insulin-stimulated glucose disposal in older males, J. Am. Geriatr. Soc., 33, 273-277, 1985.

Holt S, Heading RC, Carter DC, Prescott LF, Tothill P, Effect of gel fiber on gastric emptying and the absorption of glucose and paracetamol, Lancet , 1, 636-9, 1979.

Holt S, Gastric emptying: control and measurement, Survey of Digestive Diseases, 3, 4, 210-229, 1985.

Holt S, Observations on the relations between alcohol absorption and the rate of gastric emptying, Canadian Medical Association Journal, 124(3), 267-77, 1981.

Holt S, Skinner HA, Israel Y, Identification of alcohol abuse II, Clinical and laboratory indicators, Canadian Medical

Association Journal, 124(9), 1141-52, 1981.

Holt S, Skinner HA, Confronting Alcoholism, Canadian Medical Association Journal, 51, 8-9, 1990.

Holt S, Heeading RC, Clement J, Effects of Dietary Fiber, Gastroenterology, 80, 1611, 1981.

Holt S, Reid J, Taylor TV, Tothill P, Heading RC, Gastric emptying of solids in man, Gut, 24(4), 292-6, 1982.

Holt S, Tackling the alcohol problem: the case for secondary prevention, Journal of the South Carolina Medical Association, 85(12), 582-4, 1989.

Holt S, Identification and intervention for alcohol abuse, Journal of the South Carolina Medical Association, 85(12), 554-9, 1989.

Holt S, Smith M, Guram M, Skinner HA, Computer assessment of lifestyle in a gastroenterology clinic, Digestive Diseases and Sciences, 37, 7, 993-996, 1987.

Holt S, Over-the-counter histamine H2-receptor antagonists. How will they affect the treatment of acid-related diseases?, Drugs, 47(1), 1-11, 1994.

Holt S, Muntyan I, Likver L, Soya-Based Diets for Diabetes Mellitus, Alternative and Complementary Therapies, March/April, 1996.

Holt S, Soy: The Food of the Next Millennium: Korean Soybean Digest, Oct, 1997.

Israel Y, Orrego H, Holt S, MacDonald DW, Meema HE, Identification of alcohol abuse: thoracic fractures on routine chest X-rays as indicators of alcoholism, Alcoholism: Clinical and Experimental Research, 4, 420-2, 1980.

Jeppesen J, Facchini FS, and Reaven GM, Individuals with high total cholesterol/HDL cholesterol ratios are insulin resistant, J. Int. Med., 243, 293-298, 1998.

Jeppesen J, Hollenbeck CB, Zhou MY, Coulston AM, Jones C, Chen Y-DL, and Reaven GM, Relation between insulin resistance, hyperinsulinemia, postheparin plasma lipoprotein lipase activity, and post-prandial lipemia, Arterioscler. Thromb. Vasc. Biol., 15, 320-324, 1995.

Jeppesen J, Chen Y-DL, Zhou M-Y, Wang T, and Reaven GM, Effect of variations in oral fat and carbohydrate load on postprandial lipemia, Am. J. Clin. Nutr., 62, 1201-1205,

1995.

Kah CR, Crettax M, Insulin receptors and the molecular mechanism of insulin action, Diabetes Metab. Rev., 1, 5, 1985.

Kahn CR, Insulin action diabetogenesis and the cause of type II diabetes, Diabetes, 43, 1066, 1994.

Kemmer FW, Berger M, Exercise and diabetes mellitus: physical activity as part of daily life and its role in the treatment of diabetic patients, Int. J. Sports Med., 4, 77, 1983.

Kerciakes DJ, Myocardial infarction in the diabetic patient, Clin. Cardiol, 1985, 8:466.

Kissebah AH, Vydelingum N, Murray R, et al, Relation of body fat distribution to metabolic complications for blacks, Diabetes Care, 13, 1163, 1990.

Lee NA, Reasner CA, Beneficial effects of chromium supplementation on serum triglyceride levels in NIDDM, Diabetes Care, 17, 1449-1452, 1994.

Levi B, Werman MJ, Long-term fructose consumption accelerates glycation and several age-related variables in male rats, Journal of Nutrition, 128, 1442-1449, 1998.

Lucas CP, Estigarribia JA, Darga LL, and Reaven GM, Insulin and blood pressure in obesity, Hypertension, 7, 702-706, 1985.

Maheux P, Jeppesen J, Sheu WH, et al., Additive effects of obesity, hypertension and type 2 diabetes on insulin resistance, Hypertension, 24, 695-698, 1994.

Mau MK, Grandinetti A, Arakaki R, The insulin resistance syndrome in native Hawaiians, Diabetes Care, 20, 1376-1380, 1997.

Mayer-Davis EJ, D'Agostino R, Karter AJ, et al., Intensity and amount of physical activity in relation to insulin sensitivity, JAMA, 279, 669-674, 1998.

McGarry JD, Foster DW, Regulation of hepatic fatty acid oxidation and ketone production, Annu. Rev. Biochem., 49, 395-399, 1980.

Olefsky J, Farquhar JW, and Reaven GM, Relationship between fasting plasma insulin level and resistance to insulin-mediated glucose uptake in normal and diabetic subjects, Diabetes, 22, 507-513, 1973.

Olefsky JM, Pathogenesis of insulin resistance and hyperglycemia in non-insulin-dependent diabetes mellitus, Am. J. Med., 79, 1, 1985.

Olefsky JM, Reaven GM, and Farquhar JW, Effects of weight reduction on obesity: studies of carbohydrate and lipid metabolism, J. Clin. Invest., 53, 64-76, 1974.

Opara JU, Levine JH, The deadly quartet ñ the insulin resistance syndrome, Southern Medical Journal, 90, 1162-1168, 1997.

Poretsky L, Kalin MF, The gonadotropic function of insulin, Endocr. Rev., 8:132, 1987.

Reaven GM, Effects of differences in amount and kind of dietary carbohydrate on plasma glucose and insulin response in man, Am. J. Clin. Nutr., 32, 2568-2578, 1979.

Reaven, GM, Lerner RL, Stern MP, and Farquhar, JW, Role of insulin in endogenous hypertriglyceridemia, J. Clin. Invest., 46, 1756-1767, 1967.

Reaven GM, Pathophysiology of insulin resistance in human disease, Physiological Reviews, 75, 473-485, 1995.

Reaven GM, Banting Lecture, Role of insulin resistance in human diabetes, Diabetes, 37, 1595, 1988.

Richter EA, Ruderman NB, Schneider S, Diabetes and exercise, Am. J. Med., 70(Suppl 1), 201-205, 1981.

Robinson AM, Williamson DH, Physiological roles of ketone bodies as substrates and signals in mammalian tissues, Physiol. Rev., 60, 143-146, 1980.

Rosenthal M, Haskett WL, Solomon R, Widstrom A, and Reaven GM, Demonstration of a relationship between level of physical training and insulin-stimulated glucose utilization in normal humans, Diabetes, 32, 408-411, 1983.

Sanchez JL, et al., Role of sugars in human neutrophilic phagocytosis, American Journal of Clinical Nutrition, 26, 1180-1184, 1973.

Shen DC, Shieh, SM, Fuh, MT, Wu DA, Chen Y-DI, and Reaven GM, Resistance to insulin-stimulated glucose uptake in patients with hypertension, J. Clin. Endocrinol. Metab, 66, 580-583, 1988.

Sheu WH-H, Jeng C-Y, Shieh S-M, Fuh MM-T, Shen DD-C, Chen Y-DI, and Reaven GM, Insulin resistance and abnormal electrocardiograms in patients with high blood pressure, Am J. Hypertens, 5, 444-448, 1992.

Singh RB, Mohammed AN, Rastogi SS, et al., Current zinc intake and risk of diabetes and coronary artery disease and factors associated with insulin resistance in rural and urban populations of North India, Journal of the American College of Nutrition, 17, 564-570, 1998.

Skinner HA, Holt S, Allen BA, Haakonson NH, Correlation between medical and behavioral data in the assessment of alcoholism, Alcohol Clinical and Experimental Research, 4, 371-7, 1980.

Skinner HA, Holt S, Israel Y, Identification of alcohol abuse II, Clinical and laboratory indicators for a composite index, Canadian Medical Association Journal, 124(9), 1141-52, 1981.

Skinner HA, Holt S, Early intervention for alcohol problems, Journal of the Royal College of General Practitioners, 33, 787-91, 1983.

Skinner HA, Holt S, Schuller R, Ray J, Israel Y, Identification of alcohol abuse using laboratory tests and a history of trauma, Annals of Internal Medicine, 101(6), 847-51, 1984.

Skinner HA, Holt S, Sheu WJ, Israel Y, Clinical versus laboratory detection of alcohol abuse: the alcohol clinical index, British Medical Journal, 292(6537), 1703-8, 1986.

Su HY, Sheu WH-H, Chin H-ML, Jeng C-Y, Chen, Y-DL, and Reaven GM, Effect of weight loss on blood pressure and insulin resistance in normotensive and hypertensive obese individuals, Am. J. Hypertens, 8, 1067-1071, 1995.

Torjeson PA, Birkeland KI, Anderssen SA, et al., Lifestyle changes may reverse development of the insulin resistance syndrome, Diabetes Care, 20, 26-31, 1997.

Tornheim K, Oscillations of the glycolytic pathway and the purine nucleotide cycle, J. Theor. Biol., 79, 491, 1979.

Trevisan M, Liu J, Hahsas FB, et al., Syndrome X and mortality: A population-based study, American Journal of Epidemiology, 148, 958-966, 1998.

Vaag A, Henriksen JE, Beck-Nielsen H, Decreased insulin activation of glycogen synthase in skeletal muscles in young non-obese caucasian first-degree relatives of patients with non-insulin-dependent diabetes mellitus, J. Clin. Invest., 89, 782, 1992.

Vranic M, Berger M, Exercise and diabetes mellitus, Diabetes, 28, 147-150, 1979.

Warram JH, Martin BC, Drolewski AS, et al, Slow glucose removal rate and hyperinsulinemia precede the development of type II diabetes in the offspring of diabetic parents, Ann. Intern. Med., 113, 909-911, 1990.

Wheat LJ, Infection and diabetes, Diabetes Care, 3, 187-191, 1980.

White MF, Kahn CR, The insulin signaling System, J. Biol. Chem., 269-272, 1, 1994.

Williams KV, Korytkowski MT, Syndrome X: Pathogenesis, clinical and therapeutic aspects, Diabetes Nutrition and Metabolism, 11, 140-152. 1998.

Zavaroni I, Bonati PA, Luchetti L, Bonora E, Buonanno G, Bergonzani M, Pagliara M, Gnudi L, Butturini L, Passeri M, and Reaven GM, Habitual leisure-time physical activity is associated with differences in various risk factors for coronary artery disease, J. Int. Med., 226, 417-421, 1989.

Zavaroni I, Bonini L, Fantuzzi M, Dall'Aglio E, Passeri M, and Reaven GM, Hyperinsulinaemia, obesity, and Syndrome X, J. Int. Med., 235, 51-56, 1994.

Zavaroni I, Dall'Aglio E, Bonora E, Alpi O, Passeri M, and Reaven GM, Evidence that multiple risk factors for coronary artery disease exist in persons with abnormal glucose tolerance, Am. J. Med., 83, 609-612, 1987.

Zavaroni L, Bonini L, Gasparini P, Dall'Aglio E, Passeri M, and Reaven GM, Cigarette smokers are relatively glucose intolerant, hyperinsulinemic and dyslipidemic, Am. J. Cardiol, 73:904-905, 1994.

# BASIC RESOURCES

www.combatsyndromeX.com
Author's site

www.diabetes.org
American Diabetes Association

www.amhrt.org
American Heart Association

www.centerforpcos.bsd.uchicago.edu
Center for PCOS

www.mayohealth.org
Mayo Clinic Health Oasis

www.medscape.com
Medscape

www.ndei.org
National Diabetes Education Initiative

www.niddk.nih.gov
National Diabetes Information Clearinghouse

www.nih.gov/icd/
National Institutes of Health

www.consumer.gov/weightloss/
Partnership for Healthy Weight Management

www.syndromex.stanford.edu
Stanford University School of Medicine

www.themetabolicsyndrome.com
Author's site

www.naturesbenefit.com
Commercial sources of product

www.syndromex.tv
Educational/Practice/Research

www.wellnesspublishing.com
Educational/commercial

www.enaturalhealth.com
Education/Books

www.sindromeX.com
Educational/Spanish

www.metabolicsyndromeX.com
Educational/Products

www.enzy.com
Educational/Products

# About the Author

Stephen Holt MD is a board certified gastroenterologist and industry best-selling author from New York. He described the physiological effects of soluble fiber on upper digestive function in the Lancet in 1979 (a basis of the Glycemic Index). Dr. Holt is a frequent guest lecturer at scientific meetings and a popular media expert on therapeutics.

Other books by the author:

Holt S, *The Soy Revolution*, Dell Publishing, Random House, NY, NY, 1999 (third printing 2002).

Holt S, *The Natural Way to a Healthy Heart*, M. Evans Inc., 1999 (second printing 2002).

Holt S, *Natural Ways to Digestive Health*, M. Evans Inc., 2000 (second printing 2002).

Holt S, Comac L, *Miracle Herbs*, Carol Publishing, NJ, 1997.

Holt S, Barilla J, *The Power of Cartilage*, Kensington Publishers, NY, 1998.

Holt S, Bader D, *Natures Benefit For Pets*, Wellness Publishing.

Dr. Holts' books are available in major bookstores and on the intenet at www.wellnesspublishing.com.